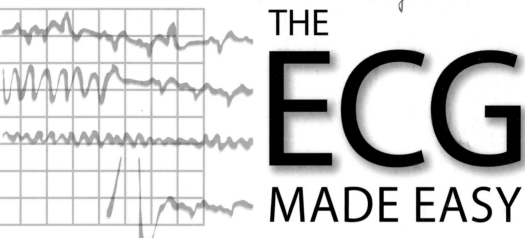

THE
ECG
MADE EASY

SEVENTH EDITION

D0898355

Commissioning Editor: Laurence Hunter
Development Editor: Hannah Kenner
Project Manager: Susan Stuart and Helius
Designer: Sarah Russell
Illustrator: Helius and Gecko Ltd
Illustration Manager: Bruce Hogarth

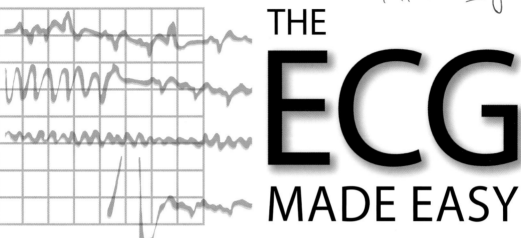

THE
ECG
MADE EASY

SEVENTH EDITION

John R. Hampton

DM MA DPhil FRCP FFPM FESC

Emeritus Professor of Cardiology
University of Nottingham
Nottingham, UK

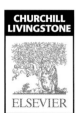

CHURCHILL LIVINGSTONE

ELSEVIER

EDINBURGH LONDON NEW YORK OXFORD PHILADELPHIA ST LOUIS SYDNEY TORONTO 2008

CHURCHILL
LIVINGSTONE
ELSEVIER

First edition 1973   Fifth edition 1997
Second edition 1980   Sixth edition 2003
Third edition 1986   Seventh edition 2008
Fourth edition 1992

Standard edition ISBN: 978-0-443-06817-1
International edition ISBN: 978-0-443-06826-3
  Reprinted 2009

British Library Cataloguing in Publication Data
A catalogue record for this book is available from the British Library

Library of Congress Cataloguing in Publication Data
A catalogue record for this book is available from the Library of Congress

Note
Knowledge and best practice in this field are constantly changing. As new research and experience broaden our knowledge, changes in practice, treatment and drug therapy may become necessary or appropriate. Readers are advised to check the most current information provided (i) on procedures featured or (ii) by the manufacturer of each product to be administered, to verify the recommended dose or formula, the method and duration of administration, and contraindications. It is the responsibility of the practitioner, relying on their own experience and knowledge of the patient, to make diagnoses, to determine dosages and the best treatment for each individual patient, and to take all appropriate safety precautions. To the fullest extent of the law, neither the Publisher nor the Author assume any liability for any injury and/or damage to persons or property arising out or related to any use of the material contained in this book.

The Publisher

Preface

The ECG Made Easy was first published in 1973, and over half a
million copies of the first six editions have been sold. The book has
been translated into German, French, Spanish, Italian, Portuguese,
Polish, Czech, Indonesian, Japanese, Russian and Turkish, and into
two Chinese languages. The aims of this edition are the same as
before: the book is not intended to be a comprehensive textbook of
electrophysiology, nor even of ECG interpretation – it is designed as
an introduction to the ECG for medical students, technicians, nurses
and paramedics. It may also provide useful revision for those who
have forgotten what they learned as students.

There really is no need for the ECG to be daunting: just as most
people drive a car without knowing much about engines, and
gardeners do not need to be botanists, most people can make full use
of the ECG without getting submerged in its complexities. This book
encourages the reader to accept that the ECG is easy to understand
and that its use is just a natural extension of taking the patient's
history and performing a physical examination.

This is the seventh edition of the book, and the most obvious
difference from the earlier editions is the change in shape that allows
12-lead ECGs to be printed across a single page. This additional

Further reading

The symbol

indicates cross-references to useful information in the book *The ECG in Practice*, 5th edn.

What the ECG is about

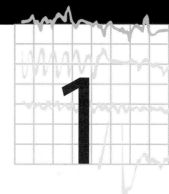

'ECG' stands for electrocardiogram, or electrocardiograph. In some countries, the abbreviation used is 'EKG'. Remember:

- By the time you have finished this book, you should be able to say *and mean* 'The ECG is easy to understand'.
- Most abnormalities of the ECG are amenable to reason.

able to be affected by

WHAT TO EXPECT FROM THE ECG

Clinical diagnosis depends mainly on a patient's history, and to a lesser extent on the physical examination. The ECG can provide evidence to support a diagnosis, and in some cases it is crucial for patient management. It is, however, important to see the ECG as a tool, and not as an end in itself.

The ECG is essential for the diagnosis, and therefore management, of abnormal cardiac rhythms. It helps with the diagnosis of the cause of chest pain, and the proper use of thrombolysis in treating myocardial infarction depends upon it. It can help with the diagnosis of the cause of breathlessness.

With practice, interpreting the ECG is a matter of pattern recognition. However, the ECG can be analysed from first principles if a few simple rules and basic facts are remembered. This chapter is about these rules and facts.

THE ELECTRICITY OF THE HEART

The contraction of any muscle is associated with electrical changes called 'depolarization', and these changes can be detected by electrodes attached to the surface of the body. Since all muscular contraction will be detected, the electrical changes associated with contraction of the heart muscle will only be clear if the patient is fully relaxed and no skeletal muscles are contracting.

Although the heart has four chambers, from the electrical point of view it can be thought of as having only two, because the two atria contract together and then the two ventricles contract together.

THE WIRING DIAGRAM OF THE HEART

The electrical discharge for each cardiac cycle normally starts in a special area of the right atrium called the 'sinoatrial (SA) node' (Fig. 1.1). Depolarization then spreads through the atrial muscle fibres. There is a delay while the depolarization spreads through another special area in the atrium, the 'atrioventricular node' (also called the 'AV node', or sometimes just 'the node'). Thereafter, the electrical discharge travels very rapidly down specialized conduction tissue, the 'bundle of His', which divides in the septum between the ventricles into right and left bundle branches. The left bundle branch itself divides into two. Within the mass of ventricular muscle, conduction spreads somewhat more slowly, through specialized tissue called 'Purkinje fibres'.

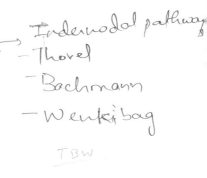

(handwritten margin notes) Internodal pathway → — Thorel — Bachmann — Wenkibag   TBW

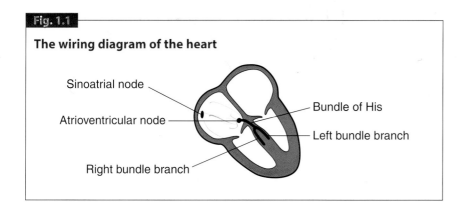

Fig. 1.1

The wiring diagram of the heart

Sinoatrial node

Atrioventricular node

Bundle of His

Left bundle branch

Right bundle branch

THE RHYTHM OF THE HEART

As we shall see later, electrical activation of the heart can sometimes begin in places other than the SA node. The word 'rhythm' is used to refer to the part of the heart which is controlling the activation sequence. The normal heart rhythm, with electrical activation beginning in the SA node, is called 'sinus rhythm'.

THE DIFFERENT PARTS OF THE ECG

The muscle mass of the atria is small compared with that of the ventricles, and so the electrical change accompanying the contraction of the atria is small. Contraction of the atria is associated with the ECG wave called 'P' (Fig. 1.2). The ventricular mass is large, and so there is a large deflection of the ECG when the ventricles are depolarized: this is called the 'QRS' complex. The 'T' wave of the ECG is associated with

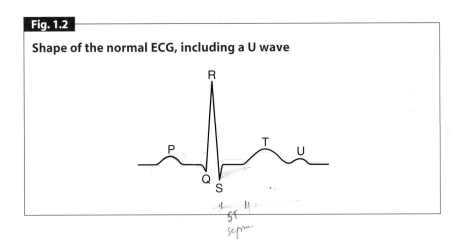

Fig. 1.2

Shape of the normal ECG, including a U wave

Fig. 1.3

Parts of the QRS complex

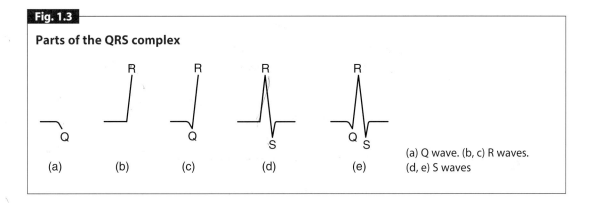

(a) Q wave. (b, c) R waves.
(d, e) S waves

the return of the ventricular mass to its resting electrical state ('repolarization').

The letters P, Q, R, S and T were selected in the early days of ECG history, and were chosen arbitrarily. The P, Q, R, S and T deflections are all called waves; the Q, R and S waves together make up a complex; and the interval between the S wave and the beginning of the T wave is called the ST 'segment'.

In some ECGs an extra wave can be seen on the end of the T wave, and this is called a U wave. Its origin is uncertain, though it may represent repolarization of the papillary muscles. If a U wave follows a normally shaped T wave it can be assumed to be normal. If it follows a flattened T wave, it may be pathological (see Ch. 4).

The different parts of the QRS complex are labelled as shown in Figure 1.3. If the first deflection is downward, it is called a Q wave (Fig. 1.3a). An upward deflection is called an R wave, regardless of whether it is preceded by a Q wave or not (Figs 1.3b and 1.3c). Any deflection below the baseline following an R wave is called an S wave, regardless of whether there has been a preceding Q wave or not (Figs 1.3d and 1.3e).

TIMES AND SPEEDS

ECG machines record changes in electrical activity by drawing a trace on a moving paper strip. ECG machines run at a standard rate of 25 mm/s and use paper with standard-sized squares. Each large square (5 mm) represents 0.2 seconds (s), i.e. 200 milliseconds (ms) (Fig. 1.4). Therefore, there are five large squares per second, and 300 per minute. So an ECG event, such as a QRS complex, occurring once per large square is occurring at a rate of 300/min. The heart rate can be calculated rapidly by remembering the sequence in Table 1.1.

Just as the length of paper between R waves gives the heart rate, so the distance between the different parts of the P–QRS–T complex shows the time taken for conduction of the electrical discharge to spread through the different parts of the heart.

Fig. 1.4

Relationship between the squares on ECG paper and time. Here, there is one QRS complex per second, so the heart rate is 60 beats/min

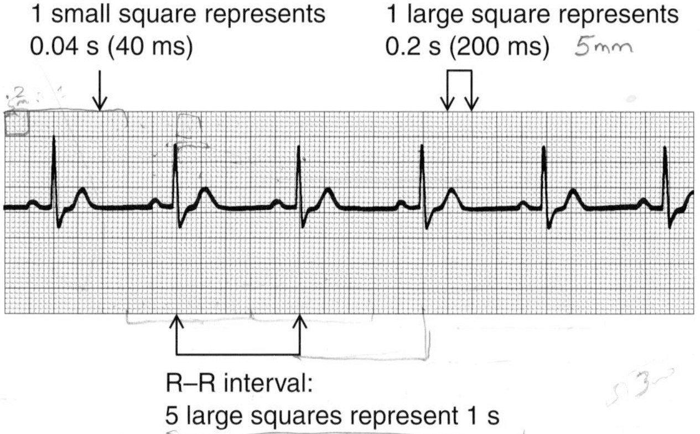

1 small square represents 0.04 s (40 ms)

1 large square represents 0.2 s (200 ms) 5mm

R–R interval: 5 large squares represent 1 s

Table 1.1 Relationship between the number of large squares between successive R waves and the heart rate

R–R interval (large squares)	Heart rate (beats/min)
1	300
2	150
3	100
4	75
5	60
6	50

Fig. 1.5

The components of the ECG complex

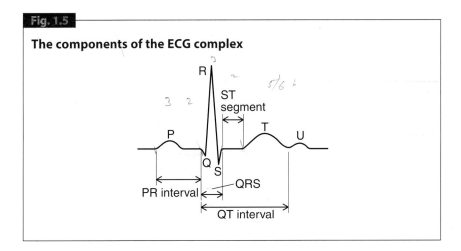

The PR interval is measured from the beginning of the P wave to the beginning of the QRS complex, and is the time taken for excitation to spread from the SA node, through the atrial muscle and the AV node, down the bundle of His and into the ventricular muscle. Logically, it should be called the PQ interval, but common usage is 'PR interval' (Fig, 1.5).

7

.12 – .2   1 small square 40ms

The normal PR interval is 120–200 ms, represented by 3–5 small squares. Most of this time is taken up by delay in the AV node (Fig. 1.6). If the PR interval is very short, either the atria have been depolarized from close to the AV node, or there is abnormally fast conduction from the atria to the ventricles.

Fig. 1.6

Normal PR interval and QRS complex

PR   *4 small (squares/bones)*   QRS   *3 small bones*
0.16 s (160 ms)   0.12 s (120 ms)

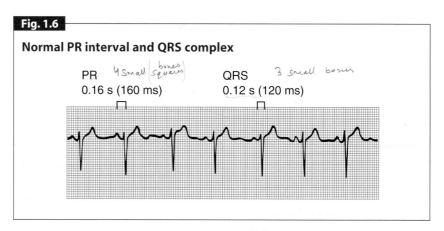

Fig. 1.7

Normal PR interval and prolonged QRS complex

PR   QRS
0.16 s (160 ms)   0.20 s (200 ms)

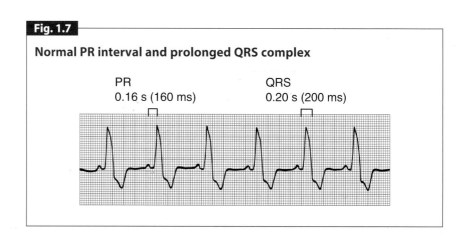

The duration of the QRS complex shows how long excitation takes to spread through the ventricles. The QRS duration is normally 120 ms (represented by three small squares) or less, but any abnormality of conduction takes longer, and causes widened QRS complexes (Fig. 1.7). Remember that the QRS complex represents depolarization, not contraction, of the ventricles – contraction is proceeding during the ECG's ST segment.

The QT interval varies with heart rate. It is prolonged in patients with some electrolyte abnormalities, and more importantly it is prolonged by some drugs. A prolonged QT interval (greater than 450 ms) may lead to ventricular tachycardia.

CALIBRATION

A limited amount of information is provided by the height of the P waves, QRS complexes and T waves, provided the machine is properly calibrated. A standard signal of 1 millivolt (mV) should move the stylus vertically 1 cm (two large squares) (Fig. 1.8), and this 'calibration' signal should be included with every record.

10mm

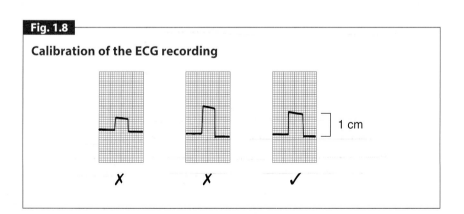

Fig. 1.8

Calibration of the ECG recording

1 cm

✗   ✗   ✓

THE ECG – ELECTRICAL PICTURES

The word 'lead' sometimes causes confusion. Sometimes it is used to mean the pieces of wire that connect the patient to the ECG recorder. Properly, a lead is an electrical picture of the heart.

The electrical signal from the heart is detected at the surface of the body through electrodes, which are joined to the ECG recorder by wires. One electrode is attached to each limb, and six to the front of the chest.

The ECG recorder compares the electrical activity detected in the different electrodes, and the electrical picture so obtained is called a 'lead'. The different comparisons 'look at' the heart from different directions. For example, when the recorder is set to 'lead I' it is comparing the electrical events detected by the electrodes attached to the right and left arms. Each lead gives a different view of the electrical activity of the heart, and so a different ECG pattern. Strictly, each ECG pattern should be called 'lead ...', but often the word 'lead' is omitted.

The ECG is made up of 12 characteristic views of the heart, six obtained from the limb leads and six from the chest leads.

THE 12-LEAD ECG

ECG interpretation is easy if you remember the directions from which the various leads look at the heart. The six 'standard' leads, which are recorded from the electrodes attached to the limbs, can be thought of as looking at the heart in a vertical plane (i.e. from the sides or the feet) (Fig. 1.9).

Leads I, II and VL look at the left lateral surface of the heart, leads III and VF at the inferior surface, and lead VR looks at the right atrium.

Fig. 1.9

The ECG patterns recorded by the six 'standard' leads

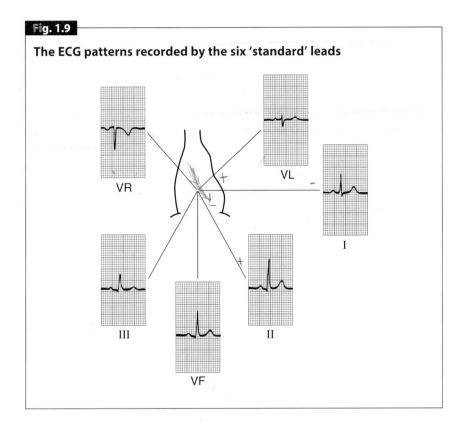

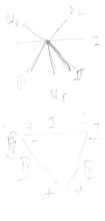

The six V leads (V₁–V₆) look at the heart in a horizontal plane, from the front and the left side. Thus leads V_1 and V_2 look at the right ventricle, V_3 and V_4 look at the septum between the ventricles and the

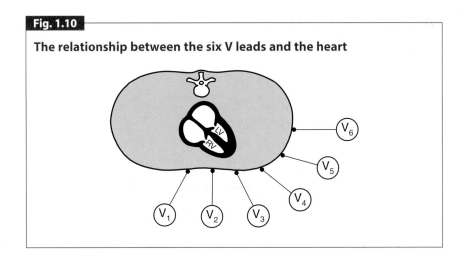

Fig. 1.10

The relationship between the six V leads and the heart

anterior wall of the left ventricle, and V_5 and V_6 look at the anterior and lateral walls of the left ventricle (Fig. 1.10).

As with the limb leads, the chest leads each show a different ECG pattern (Fig. 1.11). In each lead the pattern is characteristic, being similar in individuals who have normal hearts.

The cardiac rhythm is identified from whichever lead shows the P wave most clearly – usually lead II. When a single lead is recorded simply to show the rhythm, it is called a 'rhythm strip', but it is important not to make any diagnosis from a single lead, other than identifying the cardiac rhythm.

Fig. 1.11

The ECG patterns recorded by the chest leads

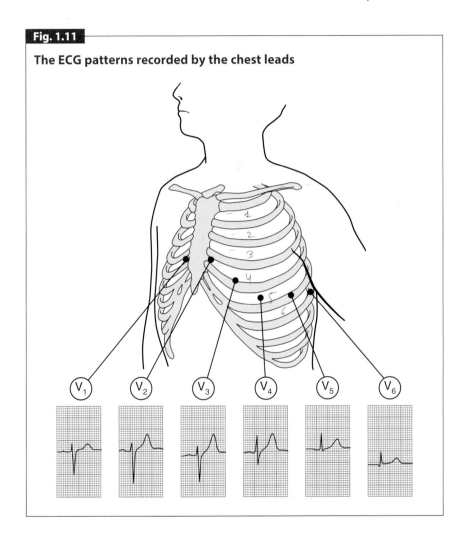

THE SHAPE OF THE QRS COMPLEX

We now need to consider why the ECG has a characteristic appearance in each lead.

THE QRS COMPLEX IN THE LIMB LEADS

The ECG machine is arranged so that when a depolarization wave spreads towards a lead the stylus moves upwards, and when it spreads away from the lead the stylus moves downwards.

Depolarization spreads through the heart in many directions at once, but the shape of the QRS complex shows the average direction in which the wave of depolarization is spreading through the ventricles (Fig. 1.12).

If the QRS complex is predominantly upward, or positive (i.e. the R wave is greater than the S wave), the depolarization is moving towards that lead (Fig. 1.12a). If predominantly downward, or negative (S wave greater than R wave), the depolarization is moving away from that lead (Fig. 1.12b). When the depolarization wave is moving at right angles to the lead, the R and S waves are of equal size (Fig. 1.12c). Q waves have a special significance, which we shall discuss later.

Fig. 1.12

Depolarization and the shape of the QRS complex

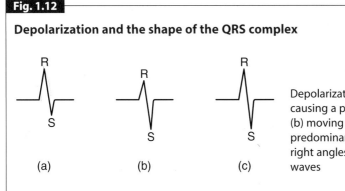

Depolarization (a) moving towards the lead, causing a predominantly upward QRS complex; (b) moving away from the lead, causing a predominantly downward QRS complex; and (c) at right angles to the lead, generating equal R and S waves

THE CARDIAC AXIS

Leads VR and II look at the heart from opposite directions. Seen from the front, the depolarization wave normally spreads through the ventricles from 11 o'clock to 5 o'clock, so the deflections in lead VR are normally mainly downward (negative) and in lead II mainly upward (positive) (Fig. 1.13).

The average direction of spread of the depolarization wave through the ventricles as seen from the front is called the 'cardiac axis'. It is useful to decide whether this axis is in a normal direction or not. The direction of the axis can be derived most easily from the QRS complex in leads I, II and III.

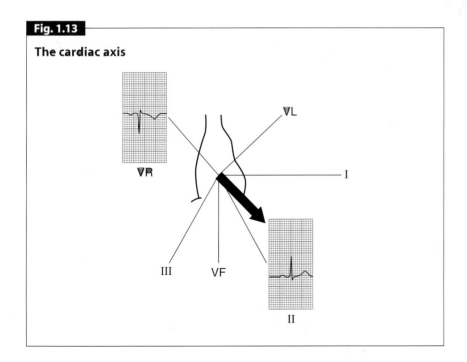

Fig. 1.13

The cardiac axis

① Estimate maximum +ve defl.

② Check Equiphasic wave
↓
Cardiac will be ①
axis
at 90° to equiphasic wave

③ Negative or inverted wave, in the lead opposite to the axis

A normal 11 o'clock–5 o'clock axis means that the depolarizing wave is spreading towards leads I, II and III and is therefore associated with a predominantly upward deflection in all these leads; the deflection will be greater in lead II than in I or III (Fig. 1.14).

When the R and S waves of the QRS complex are equal, the cardiac axis is at right angles to that lead.

If the right ventricle becomes hypertrophied, it will have more effect on the QRS complex than the left ventricle, and the average depolarization wave – the axis – will swing towards the right. The deflection in lead I becomes negative (predominantly downward) because depolarization is spreading away from it, and the deflection in lead III becomes more positive (predominantly upward) because depolarization is spreading towards it (Fig. 1.15). This is called 'right

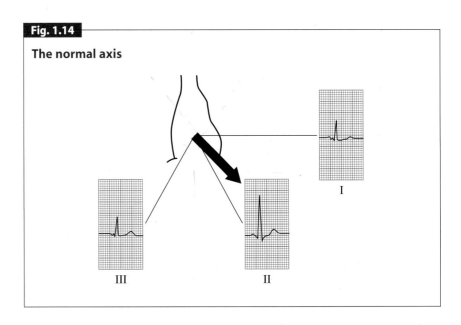

Fig. 1.14

The normal axis

III

II

I

axis deviation'. It is associated mainly with pulmonary conditions that put a strain on the right side of the heart, and with congenital heart disorders.

When the left ventricle becomes hypertrophied, it exerts more influence on the QRS complex than the right ventricle. Hence, the axis may swing to the left, and the QRS complex becomes predominantly negative in lead III (Fig. 1.16). 'Left axis deviation' is not significant until the QRS deflection is also predominantly negative in lead II. Although left axis deviation can be due to excess influence of an enlarged left ventricle, in fact this axis change is usually due to a conduction defect rather than to increased bulk of the left ventricular muscle (see Ch. 2).

Fig. 1.15

Right axis deviation

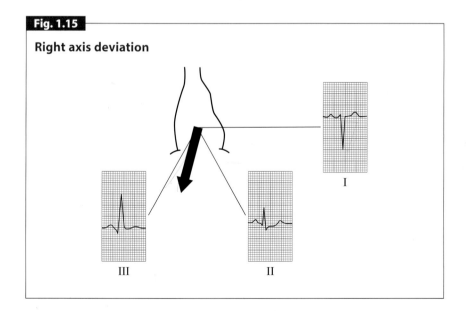

I

III   II

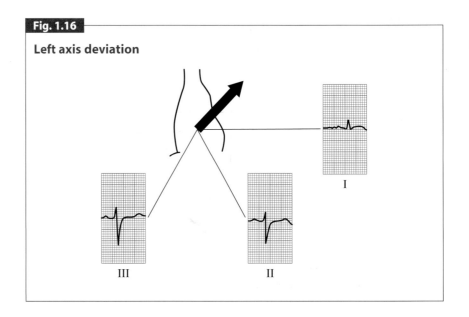

Fig. 1.16

Left axis deviation

I

III

II

The cardiac axis is sometimes measured in degrees (Fig. 1.17), though this is not clinically particularly useful. Lead I is taken as looking at the heart from 0°; lead II from +60°; lead VF from +90°; and lead III from +120°. Leads VL and VR look from −30° and −150°, respectively.

The normal cardiac axis is in the range −30° to +90°. If in lead II the S wave is greater than the R wave, the axis must be more than 90° away from lead II. In other words, it must be at a greater angle than −30°, and closer to the vertical (see Figs 1.16 and 1.17), and left axis deviation is present. Similarly, if the size of the R wave equals that of the S wave in lead I, the axis is at right angles to lead I or at +90°. This is the limit of normality towards the 'right'. If the S wave is greater than the R wave in lead I, the axis is at an angle of greater than +90°, and right axis deviation is present (Fig. 1.15).

Fig. 1.17

The cardiac axis and lead angles

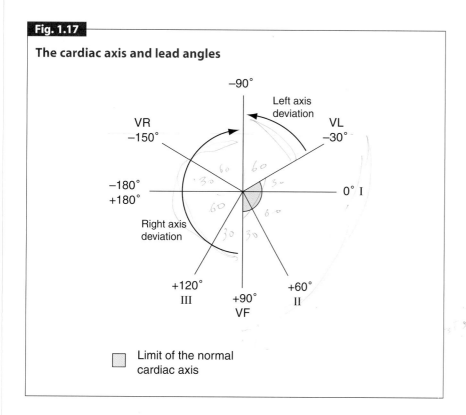

☐ Limit of the normal cardiac axis

WHY WORRY ABOUT THE CARDIAC AXIS?

Right and left axis deviation in themselves are seldom significant – minor degrees occur in tall, thin individuals and in short, fat individuals, respectively. However, the presence of axis deviation should alert you to look for other signs of right and left ventricular hypertrophy (see Ch. 4). A change in axis to the right may suggest a pulmonary embolus, and a change to the left indicates a conduction defect.

19

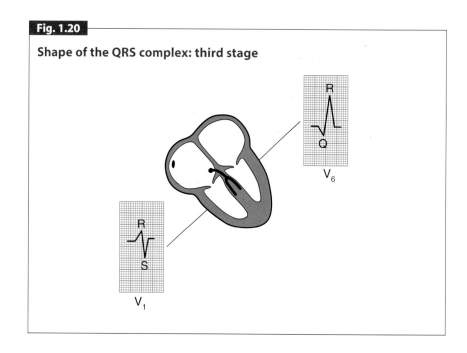

Fig. 1.20

Shape of the QRS complex: third stage

When the whole of the myocardium is depolarized the ECG trace returns to baseline (Fig. 1.20).

The QRS complex in the chest leads shows a progression from lead V_1, where it is predominantly downward, to lead V_6, where it is predominantly upward (Fig. 1.21). The 'transition point', where the R and S waves are equal, indicates the position of the interventricular septum.

WHY WORRY ABOUT THE TRANSITION POINT?

If the right ventricle is enlarged, and occupies more of the precordium than is normal, the transition point will move from its normal position of leads V_3/V_4 to leads V_4/V_5 or sometimes leads V_5/V_6. Seen from

Fig. 1.21

The ECG patterns recorded by the chest leads

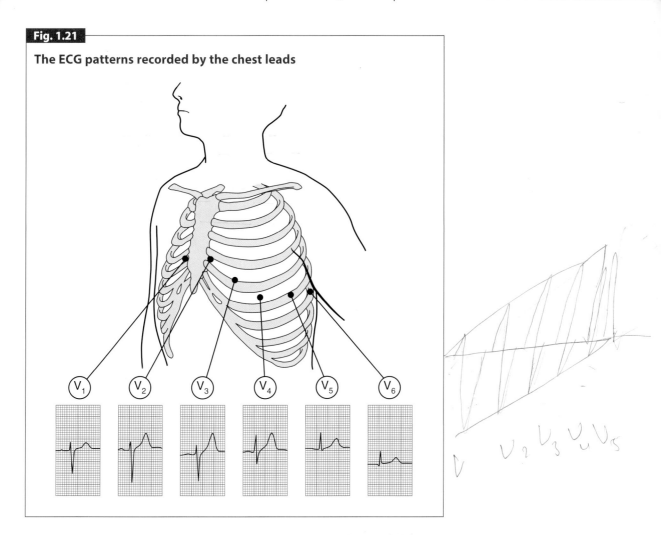

below, the heart can be thought of as having rotated in a clockwise direction. 'Clockwise rotation' in the ECG is characteristic of chronic lung disease.

MAKING A RECORDING – PRACTICAL POINTS

Now that you know what an ECG should look like, and why it looks the way it does, we need to think about the practical side of making a recording. The next series of ECGs were all recorded from a healthy subject whose 'ideal' ECG is shown in Figure 1.22.

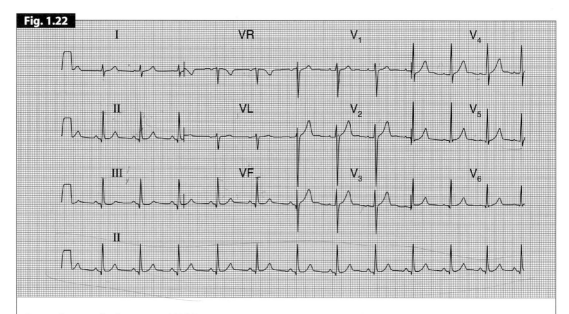

Fig. 1.22

A good record of a normal ECG

Note
- The upper three traces show the six limb leads (I, II, III, VR, VL, VF) and then the six chest leads
- The bottom trace is a 'rhythm strip', recorded from lead II (i.e. no lead changes)
- The trace is clear, with P waves, QRS complexes and T waves visible in all leads

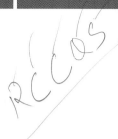

It is not necessary to remember how the six limb leads (or views of the heart) are derived by the recorder from the four electrodes attached to the limbs, but for those who like to known how it works, see Table 1.2.

The electrode attached to the right leg is used as an earth and does not contribute to any lead.

The really important thing is to make sure that the electrode marked LA is indeed attached to the left arm, RA to the right arm and so on. If the limb electrodes are wrongly attached, the 12-lead ECG will look very odd (Fig. 1.23). It is possible to work out what has happened, but it is easier to recognize that there has been a mistake, and to repeat the recording.

Table 1.2 ECG leads
Key: LA, left arm; RA, right arm; LL, left leg

Lead	Comparison of electrical activity
I	LA and RA
II	LL and RA
III	LL and LA
VR	RA and average of (LA + LL)
VL	LA and average of (RA + LL)
VF	LL and average of (LA + RA)
V_1	V_1 and average of (LA + RA + LL)
V_2	V_2 and average of (LA + RA + LL)
V_3	V_3 and average of (LA + RA + LL)
V_4	V_4 and average of (LA + RA + LL)
V_5	V_5 and average of (LA + RA + LL)
V_6	V_6 and average of (LA + RA + LL)

Fig. 1.23

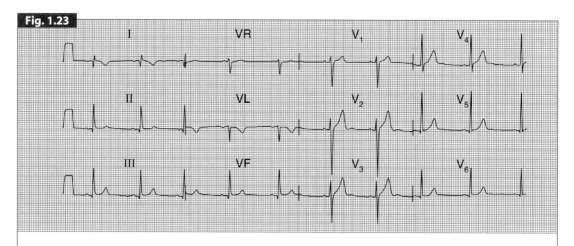

The effect of reversing the electrodes attached to the left and right arms

Note
- Compare with Figure 1.22, correctly recorded from the same patient
- Inverted P waves in lead I
- Abnormal QRS complexes and T waves in lead I
- Upright T waves in lead VR are most unusual

Reversal of the leg electrodes does not make much difference to the ECG.

The chest electrodes need to be accurately positioned, so that abnormal patterns in the V leads can be identified, and so that records taken on different occasions can be compared. Identify the second rib interspace by feeling for the sternal angle – this is the point where the manubrium and the body of the sternum meet, and there is usually a palpable ridge where the body of the sternum begins, angling

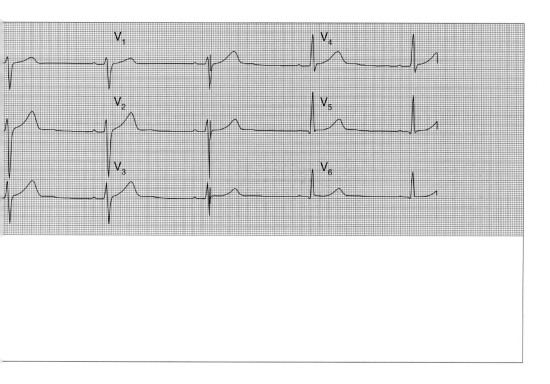

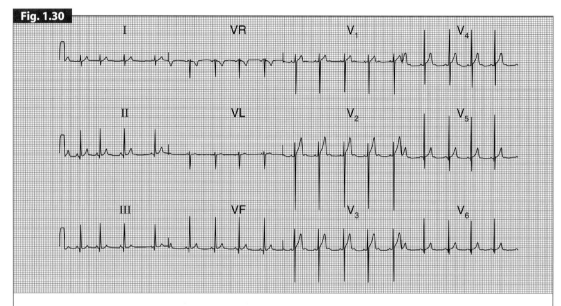

Fig. 1.30

A normal ECG recorded with a paper speed of 12.5 mm/s

Note
- A paper speed of 12.5 mm/s is slower than normal
- QRS complexes are close together, giving the impression of a rapid heart rate
- P waves, QRS complexes and T waves are all narrow and 'spiky'

ECG recorders are 'tuned' to the electrical frequency generated by heart muscle, but they will also detect the contraction of skeletal muscle. It is therefore essential that a patient is relaxed, warm, and lying comfortably – if they are moving or shivering, or have involuntary movements such as those of Parkinson's disease, the recorder will pick up a lot of muscular activity, which in extreme cases can mask the ECG (Figs 1.31 and 1.32).

So – the ECG recorder will do most of the work for you, but remember to:

- attach the electrodes to the correct limbs
- ensure good electrical contact
- check the calibration and speed settings
- get the patient comfortable and relaxed.

Then just press the button, and the recorder will automatically provide a beautiful 12-lead ECG.

Fig. 1.31

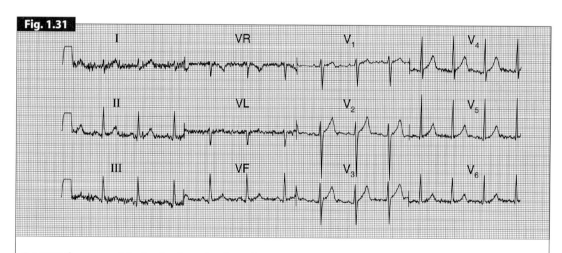

An ECG from a subject who is not relaxed

Note
- Same patient as in Fig. 1.22
- The baseline is no longer clear, and is replaced by a series of sharp irregular spikes – particularly marked in the limb leads

35

THINGS TO REMEMBER

1. The ECG results from electrical changes associated with activation first of the atria and then of the ventricles.
2. Atrial activation causes the P wave.
3. Ventricular activation causes the QRS complex. If the first deflection is downward it is a Q wave. Any upward deflection is an R wave. A downward deflection after an R wave is an S wave.

4. When the depolarization wave spreads towards a lead, the deflection is predominantly upward. When the wave spreads away from a lead, the deflection is predominantly downward.
5. The six limb leads (I, II, III, VR, VL and VF) look at the heart from the sides and the feet in a vertical plane.
6. The cardiac axis is the average direction of spread of depolarization as seen from the front, and is estimated from leads I, II and III.
7. The chest or V leads look at the heart from the front and the left side in a horizontal plane. Lead V_1 is positioned over the right ventricle, and lead V_6 over the left ventricle.
8. The septum is depolarized from the left side to the right.
9. In a normal heart the left ventricle exerts more influence on the ECG than the right ventricle.
10. Unfortunately, there are a lot of minor variations in ECGs which are consistent with perfectly normal hearts. Recognizing the limits of normality is one of the main difficulties of ECG interpretation.

ECG
IP

For more information on normal variants of the ECG, see Chapter 1

Conduction and its problems

We have already seen that electrical activation normally begins in the sinoatrial (SA) node, and that a wave of depolarization spreads outwards through the atrial muscle to the atrioventricular (AV) node, and thence down the His bundle and its branches to the ventricles. The conduction of this wave front can be delayed or blocked at any point. However, conduction problems are simple to analyse provided you keep the wiring diagram of the heart constantly in mind (Fig. 2.1).

We can think of conduction problems in the order in which the depolarization wave normally spreads: SA node → AV node → His bundle → bundle branches. Remember in all that follows that we are assuming depolarization begins in the normal way in the SA node.

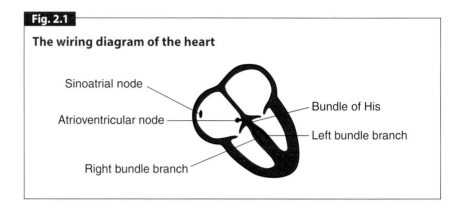

Fig. 2.1

The wiring diagram of the heart

The rhythm of the heart is best interpreted from whichever ECG lead shows the P wave most clearly. This is usually, but not always, lead II or lead V_1. You can assume that all the 'rhythm strips' in this book were recorded from one of these leads.

CONDUCTION PROBLEMS IN THE AV NODE AND HIS BUNDLE

The time taken for the spread of depolarization from the SA node to the ventricular muscle is shown by the PR interval (see Ch. 1), and is not normally greater than 0.2 s (one large square). ECG events are usually timed in milliseconds rather than seconds, so the limit of the PR interval is 200 ms.

Interference with the conduction process causes the phenomenon called 'heart block'.

FIRST DEGREE HEART BLOCK

If each wave of depolarization that originates in the SA node is conducted to the ventricles, but there is delay somewhere along the

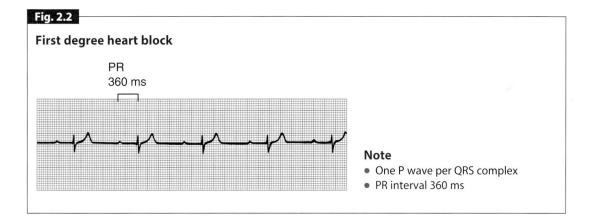

Fig. 2.2

First degree heart block

PR
360 ms

Note
- One P wave per QRS complex
- PR interval 360 ms

conduction pathway, then the PR interval is prolonged. This is called 'first degree heart block' (Fig. 2.2).

First degree heart block is not in itself important, but it may be a sign of coronary artery disease, acute rheumatic carditis, digoxin toxicity or electrolyte disturbances.

SECOND DEGREE HEART BLOCK

Sometimes excitation completely fails to pass through the AV node or the bundle of His. When this occurs *intermittently*, 'second degree heart block' is said to exist. There are three variations of this:

1. Most beats are conducted with a constant PR interval, but occasionally there is an atrial contraction without a subsequent ventricular contraction. This is called the 'Mobitz type 2' phenomenon (Fig. 2.3).
2. There may be progressive lengthening of the PR interval and then failure of conduction of an atrial beat, followed by a conducted beat with a shorter PR interval and then a repetition of this cycle. This is the 'Wenckebach' phenomenon (Fig. 2.4).

43

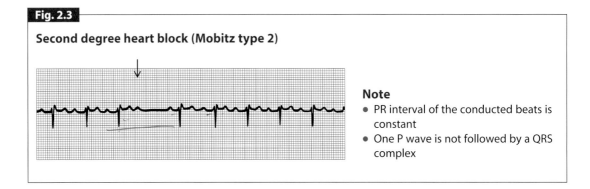

Fig. 2.3

Second degree heart block (Mobitz type 2)

Note
- PR interval of the conducted beats is constant
- One P wave is not followed by a QRS complex

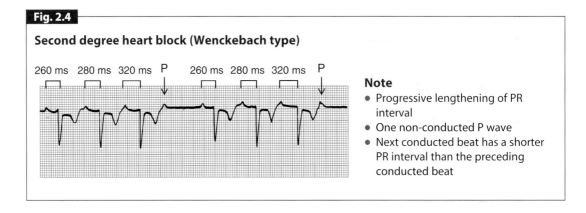

Fig. 2.4

Second degree heart block (Wenckebach type)

260 ms   280 ms   320 ms   P   260 ms   280 ms   320 ms   P

Note
- Progressive lengthening of PR interval
- One non-conducted P wave
- Next conducted beat has a shorter PR interval than the preceding conducted beat

3. There may be alternate conducted and non-conducted atrial beats (or one conducted atrial beat and then two non-conducted beats), giving twice (or three times) as many P waves as QRS complexes. This is called '2:1' ('two to one') or '3:1' ('three to one') conduction (Fig. 2.5).

It is important to remember that, as with any other rhythm, a P wave may only show itself as a distortion of a T wave (Fig. 2.6).

Fig. 2.5

Second degree heart block (2:1 type)

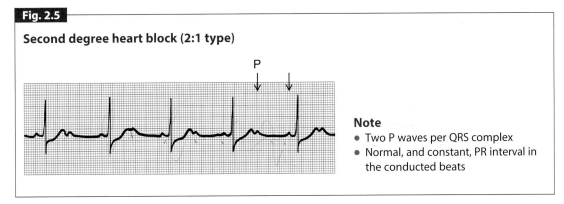

Note
- Two P waves per QRS complex
- Normal, and constant, PR interval in the conducted beats

Fig. 2.6

Second degree heart block (2:1 type)

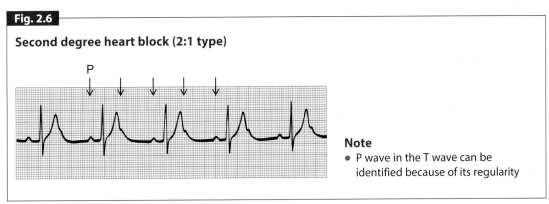

Note
- P wave in the T wave can be identified because of its regularity

The underlying causes of second degree heart block are the same as those of first degree block. The Wenckebach phenomenon is usually benign, but Mobitz type 2 block and 2:1 block may herald 'complete,' or 'third degree', heart block.

THIRD DEGREE HEART BLOCK

Complete heart block (third degree block) is said to occur when atrial contraction is normal but no beats are conducted to the ventricles (Fig. 2.7). When this occurs the ventricles are excited by a slow 'escape mechanism' (see Ch. 3), from a depolarizing focus within the ventricular muscle.

Complete block is not always immediately obvious in a 12-lead ECG, where there may be only a few QRS complexes per lead (e.g. see Fig. 2.8). You have to look at the PR interval in all the leads to see that there is no consistency.

Complete heart block may occur as an acute phenomenon in patients with myocardial infarction (when it is usually transient) or it may be a chronic state, usually due to fibrosis around the bundle of His. It may also be caused by the block of both bundle branches.

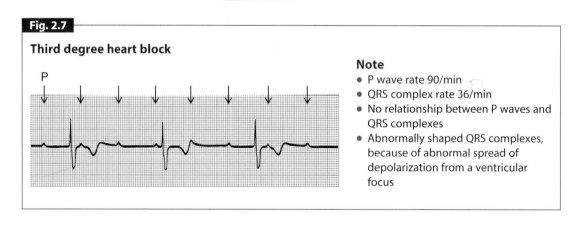

Fig. 2.7

Third degree heart block

P

Note
- P wave rate 90/min
- QRS complex rate 36/min
- No relationship between P waves and QRS complexes
- Abnormally shaped QRS complexes, because of abnormal spread of depolarization from a ventricular focus

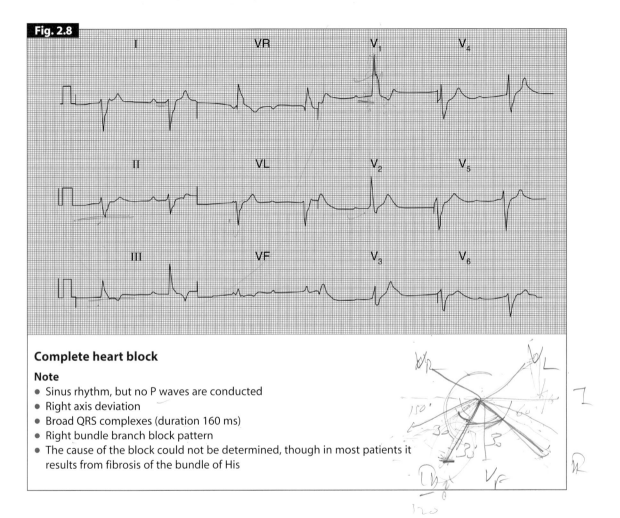

Fig. 2.8

Complete heart block

Note

- Sinus rhythm, but no P waves are conducted
- Right axis deviation
- Broad QRS complexes (duration 160 ms)
- Right bundle branch block pattern
- The cause of the block could not be determined, though in most patients it results from fibrosis of the bundle of His

CONDUCTION PROBLEMS IN THE RIGHT AND LEFT BUNDLE BRANCHES – BUNDLE BRANCH BLOCK

If the depolarization wave reaches the interventricular septum normally, the interval between the beginning of the P wave and the first deflection in the QRS complex (the PR interval) will be normal. However, if there is abnormal conduction through either the right or left bundle branches ('bundle branch block') there will be a delay in the depolarization of part of the ventricular muscle. The extra time taken for depolarization of the whole of the ventricular muscle causes widening of the QRS complex.

In the normal heart, the time taken for the depolarization wave to spread from the interventricular septum to the furthest part of the ventricles is less than 120 ms, represented by three small squares of ECG paper. If the QRS complex duration is greater than 120 ms, then conduction within the ventricles must have occurred by an abnormal and therefore slower pathway.

Although a wide QRS complex can indicate bundle branch block, widening also occurs if depolarization begins within the ventricular muscle itself (see Ch. 3). Remember that in sinus rhythm with bundle branch block, normal P waves are present with a constant PR interval. We shall see that this is not the case with rhythms beginning in the ventricles.

Block of both bundle branches has the same effect as block of the His bundle, and causes complete (third degree) heart block.

Right bundle branch block (RBBB) often indicates problems in the right side of the heart, but RBBB patterns with a QRS complex of normal duration are quite common in healthy people.

Left bundle branch block (LBBB) is always an indication of heart disease, usually of the left side. It is important to recognize that bundle branch block is present, because LBBB prevents any further interpretation of the cardiogram, and RBBB can make interpretation difficult.

The mechanism underlying the ECG patterns of RBBB and LBBB can be worked out from first principles. Remember (see Ch. 1):

- The septum is normally depolarized from left to right.
- The left ventricle, having the greater muscle mass, exerts more influence on the ECG than does the right ventricle.
- Excitation spreading towards a lead causes an upward deflection within the ECG.

RIGHT BUNDLE BRANCH BLOCK

In RBBB, no conduction occurs down the right bundle branch but the septum is depolarized from the left side as usual, causing an R wave in a right ventricular lead (V_1) and a small Q wave in a left ventricular lead (V_6) (Fig. 2.9).

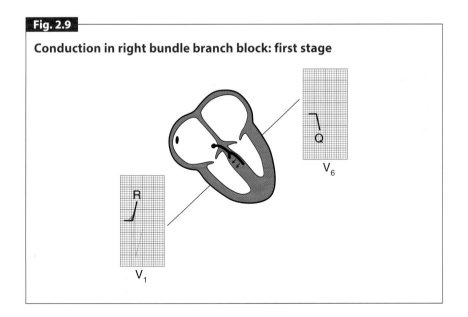

Fig. 2.9

Conduction in right bundle branch block: first stage

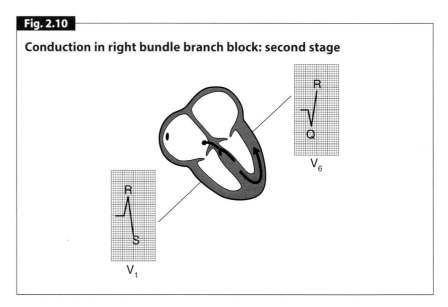

Fig. 2.10

Conduction in right bundle branch block: second stage

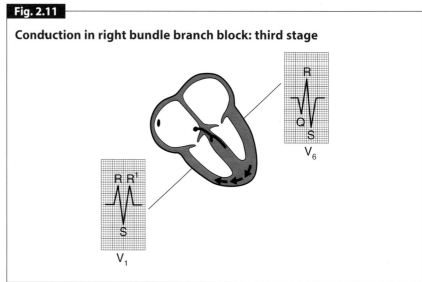

Fig. 2.11

Conduction in right bundle branch block: third stage

Fig. 2.16

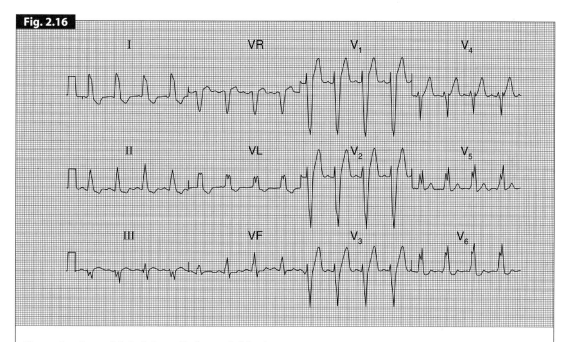

Sinus rhythm with left bundle branch block

Note

- Sinus rhythm, rate 100/min
- Normal PR interval
- Normal cardiac axis
- Wide QRS complexes (160 ms)
- M pattern in the QRS complexes, best seen in leads I, VL, V_5, V_6
- Inverted T waves in leads I, II, VL

CONDUCTION PROBLEMS IN THE DISTAL PARTS OF THE LEFT BUNDLE BRANCH

At this point it is worth considering in a little more detail the anatomy of the branches of the His bundle. The right bundle branch has no main divisions but the left bundle branch has two – the anterior and posterior 'fascicles'. The depolarization wave therefore spreads into the ventricles by three pathways (Fig. 2.17).

The cardiac axis (see Ch. 1) depends on the average direction of depolarization of the ventricles. Since the left ventricle contains more muscle than the right, it has more influence on the cardiac axis (Fig. 2.18).

If the anterior fascicle of the left bundle branch fails to conduct, the left ventricle has to be depolarized through the posterior fascicle and so the cardiac axis rotates upwards (Fig. 2.19).

Fig. 2.17

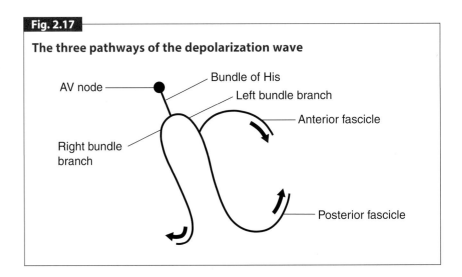

The three pathways of the depolarization wave

AV node — Bundle of His
Left bundle branch
Anterior fascicle
Right bundle branch
Posterior fascicle

Fig. 2.18

Effect of normal conduction on the cardiac axis

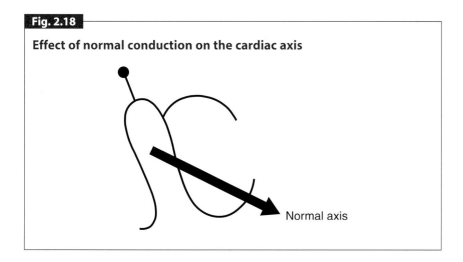

Normal axis

Fig. 2.19

Effect of left anterior fascicular block on the cardiac axis

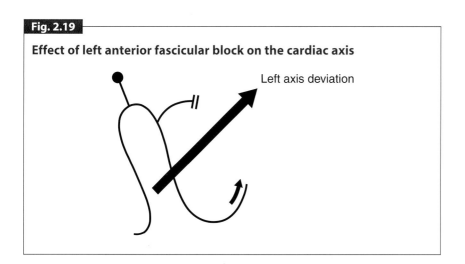

Left axis deviation

Left axis deviation is therefore due to left anterior fascicular block, or 'left anterior hemiblock' (Fig. 2.20).

The posterior fascicle of the left bundle is not often selectively blocked, but if this does occur the ECG shows right axis deviation.

When the right bundle branch is blocked, the cardiac axis usually remains normal, because there is normal depolarization of the left ventricle with its large muscle mass (Fig. 2.21).

However, if both the right bundle branch and the left anterior fascicle are blocked, the ECG shows RBBB and left axis deviation (Fig. 2.22). This is sometimes called 'bifascicular block', and this

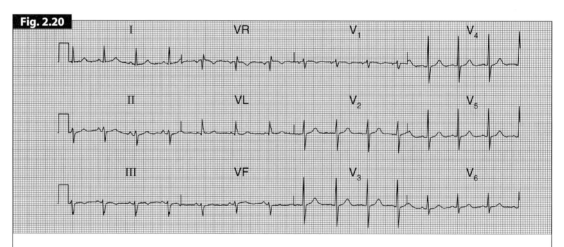

Fig. 2.20

Sinus rhythm with left axis deviation (otherwise normal)

Note
- Sinus rhythm, rate 80/min
- Left axis deviation: QRS complex upright in lead I, but downward (dominant S wave) in leads II and III
- Normal QRS complexes, ST segments and T waves

Fig. 2.21

Lack of effect of right bundle branch block (RBBB) on the cardiac axis

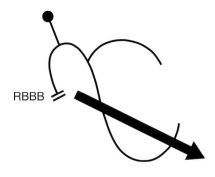

RBBB

Fig. 2.22

Effect of right bundle branch block (RBBB) and left anterior hemiblock on the cardiac axis

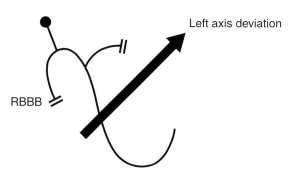

Left axis deviation

RBBB

particular ECG pattern obviously indicates widespread damage to the conducting system (Fig. 2.23).

If the right bundle branch and both fascicles of the left bundle branch are blocked, complete heart block occurs just as if the main His bundle had failed to conduct.

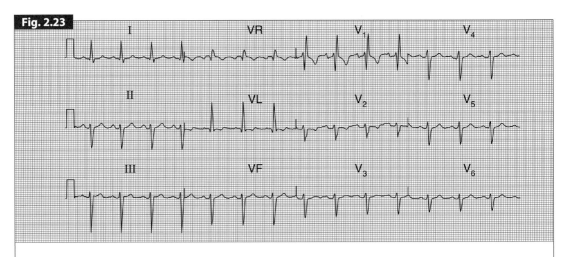

Fig. 2.23

Bifascicular block

Note
- Sinus rhythm, rate 90/min
- Left axis deviation (dominant S wave in leads II and III)
- Right bundle branch block (RSR[1] pattern in lead V_1, and deep wide S wave in lead V_6)

WHAT TO DO

Always remember that it is the patient who should be treated, not the ECG. Relief of symptoms always comes first. However, some general points can be made about the action that might be taken if the ECG shows conduction abnormalities.

First degree block

- Often seen in normal people.
- Think about acute myocardial infarction and acute rheumatic fever as possible causes.
- No specific action needed.

Second degree block

- Usually indicates heart disease; often seen in acute myocardial infarction.
- Mobitz type 2 and Wenckebach block do not need specific treatment.
- 2:1, 3:1 or 4:1 block may indicate a need for temporary or permanent pacing, especially if the ventricular rate is slow.

Third degree block

- Always indicates conducting tissue disease – more often fibrosis than ischaemic.
- Consider a temporary or permanent pacemaker.

Right bundle branch block

- Think about an atrial septal defect.
- No specific treatment.

Left bundle branch block

- Think about aortic stenosis and ischaemic disease.
- If the patient is asymptomatic, no action is needed.
- If the patient has recently had severe chest pain, LBBB may indicate an acute myocardial infarction, and thrombolysis should be considered.

Left axis deviation

- Think about left ventricular hypertrophy and its causes.
- No action needed.

Left axis deviation and right bundle branch block

- Indicates severe conducting tissue disease.
- No specific treatment needed.
- Pacemaker required if the patient has symptoms suggestive of intermittent complete heart block.

THINGS TO REMEMBER

1. Depolarization normally begins in the SA node, and spreads to the ventricles via the AV node, the His bundle, the right and left branches of the His bundle, and the anterior and posterior fascicles of the left bundle branch.
2. A conduction abnormality can develop at any of these points.
3. Conduction problems in the AV node and His bundle may be partial (first and second degree block) or complete (third degree block).

4. If conduction is normal through the AV node, the His bundle and one of its branches, but is abnormal in the other branch, bundle branch block exists and the QRS complex is wide.
5. The ECG pattern of RBBB and LBBB can be worked out if you remember that:
   — the septum is depolarized first from left to right
   — lead V_1 looks at the right ventricle and lead V_6 at the left ventricle
   — when depolarization spreads towards an electrode the stylus moves upwards.
6. If you can't remember all this, remember that RBBB has an RSR[1] pattern in lead V_1, while LBBB has a letter 'M' pattern in lead V_6.
7. Block of the anterior division or fascicle of the left bundle branch causes left axis deviation.

For more about conduction problems, see pp. 134–149

For information on the treatment of conduction problems with pacemakers, see pp. 283–307

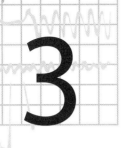

3

The rhythm of the heart

So far we have only considered the spread of depolarization that follows the normal activation of the sinoatrial (SA) node. When depolarization begins in the SA node the heart is said to be in sinus rhythm. Depolarization can, however, begin in other places. Then the rhythm is named after the part of the heart where the depolarization sequence originates, and an 'arrhythmia' is said to be present.

When attempting to analyse a cardiac rhythm remember:

- Atrial contraction is associated with the P wave of the ECG.
- Ventricular contraction is associated with the QRS complex.
- Atrial contraction normally precedes ventricular contraction, and there is normally one atrial contraction per ventricular contraction (i.e. there should be as many P waves as there are QRS complexes).

The keys to rhythm abnormalities are:

- The P waves – can you find them? Look for the lead in which they are most obvious.
- The relationship betwen the P waves and the QRS complexes – there should be one P wave per QRS complex.
- The width of the QRS complexes (should be 120 ms or less).
- Because an arrhythmia should be identified from the lead in which the P waves can be seen most easily, full 12-lead ECGs are better than rhythm strips.

THE INTRINSIC RHYTHMICITY OF THE HEART

Most parts of the heart can depolarize spontaneously and rhythmically, and the rate of contraction of the ventricles will be controlled by the part of the heart that is depolarizing most frequently.

The stars in the figures in this chapter indicate the part of the heart where the activation sequence began. The SA node normally has the highest frequency of discharge. Therefore the rate of contraction of the ventricles will equal the rate of discharge of the SA node. The rate of discharge of the SA node is influenced by the vagus nerves, and also by reflexes originating in the lungs. Changes in heart rate associated with respiration are normally seen in young people, and this is called 'sinus arrhythmia' (Fig. 3.1).

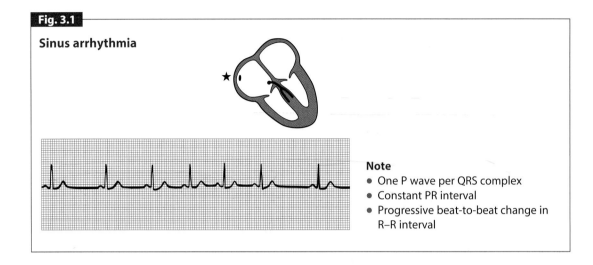

Fig. 3.1

Sinus arrhythmia

Note
- One P wave per QRS complex
- Constant PR interval
- Progressive beat-to-beat change in R–R interval

A slow sinus rhythm ('sinus bradycardia') can be associated with athletic training, fainting attacks, hypothermia or myxoedema, and is also often seen immediately after a heart attack. A fast sinus rhythm ('sinus tachycardia') can be associated with exercise, fear, pain, haemorrhage or thyrotoxicosis. There is no particular rate that is called 'bradycardia' or 'tachycardia' – these are merely descriptive terms.

ABNORMAL RHYTHMS

Abnormal cardiac rhythms can begin in one of three places (Fig. 3.2): the atrial muscle; the region around the atrioventricular (AV) node (this rhythm is called 'nodal' or, more properly, 'junctional'); or the ventricular muscle. Although Figure 3.2 suggests that electrical activation might begin at specific points within the atrial and ventricular muscles, abnormal rhythms can begin anywhere within the atria or ventricles.

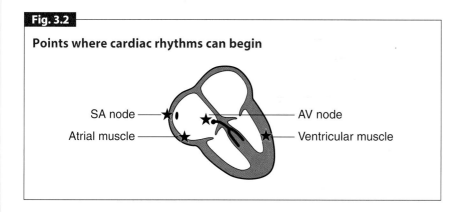

Fig. 3.2

Points where cardiac rhythms can begin

SA node

Atrial muscle

AV node

Ventricular muscle

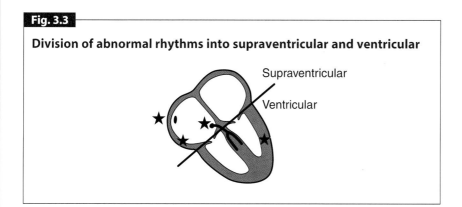

Fig. 3.3

Division of abnormal rhythms into supraventricular and ventricular

Supraventricular

Ventricular

Sinus rhythm, atrial rhythm, and junctional rhythm together constitute the 'supraventricular' rhythms (Fig. 3.3). In the supraventricular rhythms, the depolarization wave spreads to the ventricles in the normal way via the His bundle and its branches (Fig. 3.4). The QRS complex is therefore normal, and is the same whether depolarization was initiated by the SA node, the atrial muscle, or the junctional region.

These slow and protective rhythms are called 'escape rhythms', because they occur when secondary sites for initiating depolarization escape from their normal inhibition by the more active SA node.

Escape rhythms are not primary disorders, but are the response to problems higher in the conducting pathway. They are commonly seen in the acute phase of a heart attack, when they may be associated with sinus bradycardia. It is important not to try to suppress an escape rhythm, because without it the heart might stop altogether.

ATRIAL ESCAPE

If the rate of depolarization of the SA node slows down and a focus in the atrium takes over control of the heart, the rhythm is described as 'atrial escape' (Fig. 3.6). Atrial escape beats can occur singly.

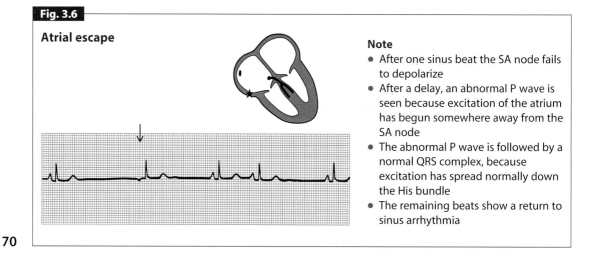

Fig. 3.6

Atrial escape

Note
- After one sinus beat the SA node fails to depolarize
- After a delay, an abnormal P wave is seen because excitation of the atrium has begun somewhere away from the SA node
- The abnormal P wave is followed by a normal QRS complex, because excitation has spread normally down the His bundle
- The remaining beats show a return to sinus arrhythmia

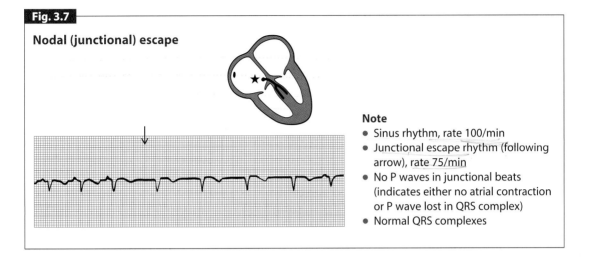

Fig. 3.7

Nodal (junctional) escape

Note
- Sinus rhythm, rate 100/min
- Junctional escape rhythm (following arrow), rate 75/min
- No P waves in junctional beats (indicates either no atrial contraction or P wave lost in QRS complex)
- Normal QRS complexes

NODAL (JUNCTIONAL) ESCAPE

If the region around the AV node takes over as the focus of depolarization, the rhythm is called 'nodal', or more properly, 'junctional' escape (Fig. 3.7).

VENTRICULAR ESCAPE

'Ventricular escape' is most commonly seen when conduction between the atria and ventricles is interrupted by complete heart block (Fig. 3.8).

Ventricular escape rhythms can occur without complete heart block, and ventricular escape beats can be single (Fig. 3.9).

The rhythm of the heart can occasionally be controlled by a ventricular focus with an intrinsic frequency of discharge faster than that seen in complete heart block. This rhythm is called 'accelerated idioventricular rhythm' (Fig. 3.10), and is often associated with acute myocardial infarction. Although the appearance of the ECG is similar

Fig. 3.8

Complete heart block

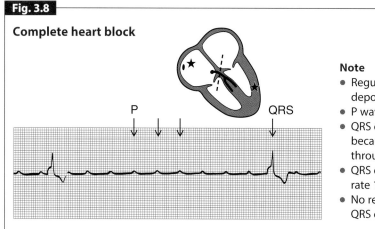

P   QRS

Note
- Regular P waves (normal atrial depolarization)
- P wave rate 145/min
- QRS complexes highly abnormal because of abnormal conduction through ventricular muscle
- QRS complex (ventricular escape) rate 15/min
- No relationship between P waves and QRS complexes

Fig. 3.9

Ventricular escape

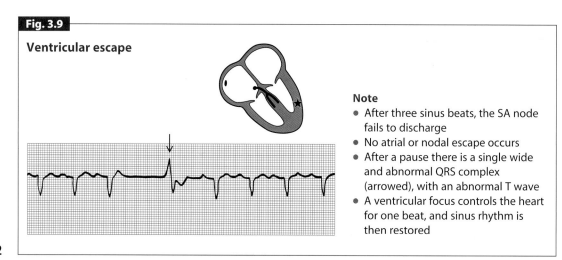

Note
- After three sinus beats, the SA node fails to discharge
- No atrial or nodal escape occurs
- After a pause there is a single wide and abnormal QRS complex (arrowed), with an abnormal T wave
- A ventricular focus controls the heart for one beat, and sinus rhythm is then restored

Fig. 3.10

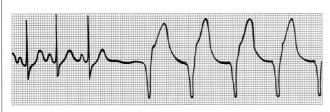

Accelerated idioventricular rhythm

Note
- After three sinus beats, the SA node fails to depolarize
- An escape focus in the ventricle takes over, causing a regular rhythm of 75/min with wide QRS complexes and abnormal T waves

to that of ventricular tachycardia (described later), accelerated idioventricular rhythm is benign and should not be treated. Ventricular tachycardia should not be diagnosed unless the heart rate exceeds 120/min.

EXTRASYSTOLES

Any part of the heart can depolarize earlier than it should, and the accompanying heartbeat is called an extrasystole. The term 'ectopic' is sometimes used to indicate that depolarization originated in an abnormal location, and the term 'premature contraction' means the same thing.

The ECG appearance of an extrasystole arising in either the atrial muscle, the junctional or nodal region, or the ventricular muscle, is the same as that of the corresponding escape beat – the difference is that an extrasystole comes early and an escape beat comes late.

Atrial extrasystoles have abnormal P waves (Fig. 3.11). In a junctional extrasystole either there is no P wave at all, or it appears

73

Fig. 3.11

Atrial and junctional (nodal) extrasystoles

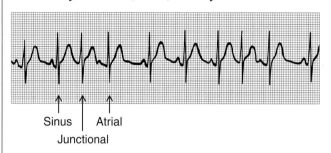

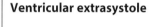

Sinus | Atrial

Junctional

Note

- This record shows sinus rhythm with junctional and atrial extrasystoles
- A junctional extrasystole has no P wave
- An atrial extrasystole has an abnormally shaped P wave
- Sinus, junctional and atrial beats have identical QRS complexes – conduction in and beyond the bundle of His is normal

Fig. 3.12

Ventricular extrasystole

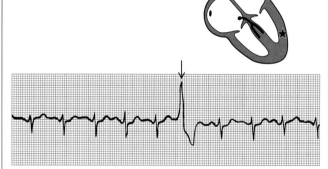

R on T phenomenon:

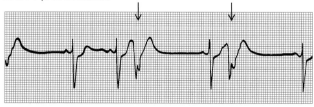

Note

- The upper trace shows five sinus beats, then an early beat with a wide QRS complex and an abnormal T wave: this is a ventricular extrasystole (arrowed)
- In the lower trace, the ventricular extrasystoles occur (arrowed) at the peak of the T waves of the preceding sinus beats: this is the 'R on T' phenomenon

immediately before or immediately after the QRS complex (Fig. 3.11). The QRS complexes of atrial and junctional extrasystoles are, of course, the same as those of sinus rhythm.

Ventricular extrasystoles, however, have abnormal QRS complexes, which are typically wide but can be of almost any shape (Fig. 3.12). Ventricular extrasystoles are common and are usually of no importance. However, when they occur early in the T wave of a preceding beat they can induce ventricular fibrillation (described later), and are thus potentially dangerous.

It may, however, not be as easy as this, particularly if a beat of supraventricular origin is conducted abnormally to the ventricles (bundle branch block, see Ch. 2). It is advisable to get into the habit of asking five questions every time an ECG is being analysed:

1. Does an early QRS complex follow an early P wave? If so, it must be an atrial extrasystole.
2. Can a P wave be seen anywhere? A junctional extrasystole may cause the appearance of a P wave very close to, and even after, the QRS complex because excitation is conducted both to the atria and to the ventricles.
3. Is the QRS complex the same shape throughout (i.e. has it the same initial direction of deflection as the normal beat, and has it the same duration)? Supraventricular beats look the same; ventricular beats look different.
4. Is the T wave the same way up as in the normal beat? In supraventricular beats, it is the same way up; in ventricular beats, it is inverted.
5. Does the next P wave after the extrasystole appear at an expected time? In both supraventricular and ventricular extrasystoles there is a ('compensatory') pause before the next heartbeat, but a supraventricular extrasystole usually upsets the normal periodicity of the SA node, so that the next SA node discharge (and P wave) comes late.

The effects of supraventricular and ventricular extrasystoles on the following P wave are as follows:

- A supraventricular extrasystole resets the P wave cycle (Fig. 3.13).
- A ventricular extrasystole, on the other hand, does not affect the SA node, so the next P wave appears at the predicted time (Fig. 3.14).

Fig. 3.13

Supraventricular extrasystole

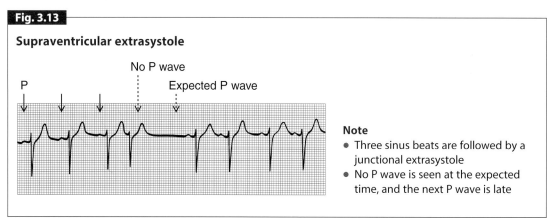

No P wave

P   Expected P wave

Note
- Three sinus beats are followed by a junctional extrasystole
- No P wave is seen at the expected time, and the next P wave is late

Fig. 3.14

Ventricular extrasystole

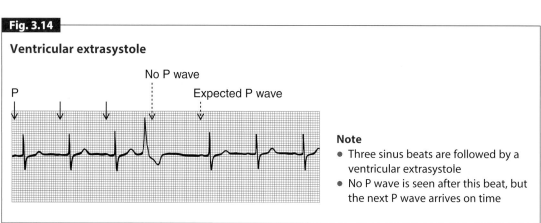

No P wave

P   Expected P wave

Note
- Three sinus beats are followed by a ventricular extrasystole
- No P wave is seen after this beat, but the next P wave arrives on time

THE TACHYCARDIAS – THE FAST RHYTHMS

Foci in the atria, the junctional (AV nodal) region, and the ventricles may depolarize repeatedly, causing a sustained tachycardia. The criteria already described can be used to decide the origin of the arrhythmia, and as before the most important thing is to try to identify a P wave. When a tachycardia occurs intermittently, it is called 'paroxysmal': this is a clinical description, and is not related to any specific ECG pattern.

SUPRAVENTRICULAR TACHYCARDIAS

Atrial tachycardia (abnormal focus in the atrium)

In atrial tachycardia, the atria depolarize faster than 150/min (Fig. 3.15).

Fig. 3.15

Atrial tachycardia

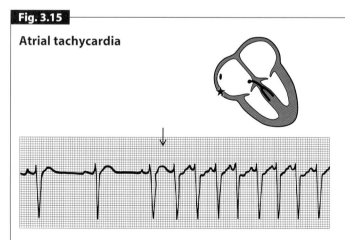

Note
- After three sinus beats, atrial tachycardia develops at a rate of 150/min
- P waves can be seen superimposed on the T waves of the preceding beats
- The QRS complexes have the same shape as those of the sinus beats

The AV node cannot conduct atrial rates of discharge greater than about 200/min. If the atrial rate is faster than this, 'atrioventricular block' occurs, with some P waves not followed by QRS complexes. The difference between this sort of atrioventricular block and second degree heart block is that in atrioventricular block associated with a tachycardia the AV node is functioning properly – it is preventing the ventricles from being activated at a fast (and therefore inefficient) rate. In first, second or third degree block associated with sinus rhythm the AV node and/or the His bundle are not conducting normally.

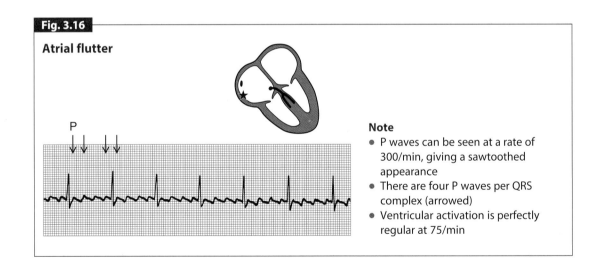

Fig. 3.16

Atrial flutter

P

Note
- P waves can be seen at a rate of 300/min, giving a sawtoothed appearance
- There are four P waves per QRS complex (arrowed)
- Ventricular activation is perfectly regular at 75/min

Atrial flutter

When the atrial rate is greater than 250/min, and there is no flat baseline between the P waves, 'atrial flutter' is present (Fig. 3.16).

When atrial tachycardia or atrial flutter is associated with 2:1 block, you need to look carefully to recognize the extra P waves (Fig. 3.17). A narrow complex tachycardia with a ventricular rate of about 125/min should always alert you to the possibility of atrial flutter with 2:1 block.

Any arrhythmia should be identified from the lead in which P waves can most easily be seen. In the record in Figure 3.18, atrial flutter is most easily seen in lead II, but it is also obvious in leads VR and VF.

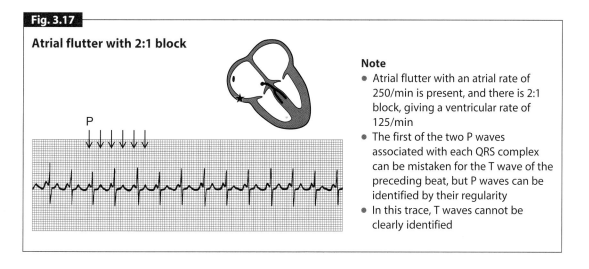

Fig. 3.17

Atrial flutter with 2:1 block

P

Note
- Atrial flutter with an atrial rate of 250/min is present, and there is 2:1 block, giving a ventricular rate of 125/min
- The first of the two P waves associated with each QRS complex can be mistaken for the T wave of the preceding beat, but P waves can be identified by their regularity
- In this trace, T waves cannot be clearly identified

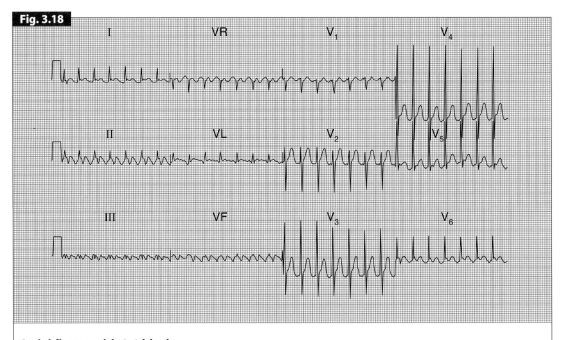

Fig. 3.18

Atrial flutter with 2:1 block

Note

- P waves at just over 300/min (most easily seen in leads II and VR)
- Regular QRS complexes, rate 160/min
- Narrow QRS complexes of normal shape
- Normal T waves (best seen in the V leads; in the limb leads it is difficult to distinguish between T and P waves)

Junctional (nodal) tachycardia

If the area around the AV node depolarizes frequently, the P waves may be seen very close to the QRS complexes, or may not be seen at all (Fig. 3.19). The QRS complex is of normal shape because, as with the other supraventricular arrhythmias, the ventricles are activated via the bundle of His in the normal way.

The 12-lead ECG in Figure 3.20 shows that in a junctional tachycardia no P waves can be seen in any lead.

Fig. 3.19

Junctional (nodal) tachycardia

Junctional tachycardia:

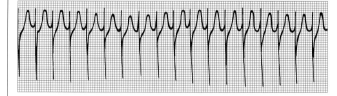

Sinus rhythm:

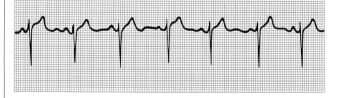

Note
- In the upper trace there are no P waves, and the QRS complexes are completely regular
- The lower trace is from the same patient, in sinus rhythm. The QRS complexes have essentially the same shape as those of the junctional tachycardia

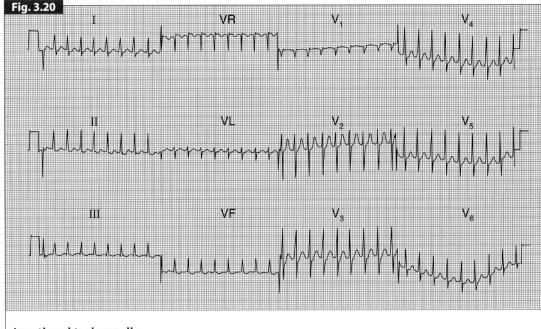

Fig. 3.20

Junctional tachycardia

Note
- No P waves
- Regular QRS complexes, rate 200/min
- Narrow QRS complexes of normal shape
- Normal T waves

Carotid sinus pressure

Carotid sinus pressure may have a useful therapeutic effect on supraventricular tachycardias, and is always worth trying because it may make the nature of the arrhythmia more obvious (Fig. 3.21). Carotid sinus pressure activates a reflex that leads to vagal stimulation of the SA and AV nodes. This causes a reduction of the frequency of discharge of the SA node, and an increase in the delay of conduction in the AV node. It is the latter which is important in the diagnosis and treatment of arrhythmias. Carotid sinus pressure slows the ventricular rate in some supraventricular arrhythmias and completely abolishes others, but it has no effect on ventricular arrhythmias.

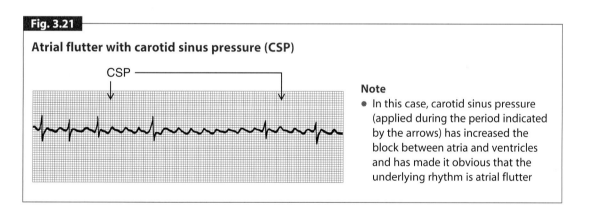

Fig. 3.21

Atrial flutter with carotid sinus pressure (CSP)

CSP

Note
- In this case, carotid sinus pressure (applied during the period indicated by the arrows) has increased the block between atria and ventricles and has made it obvious that the underlying rhythm is atrial flutter

VENTRICULAR TACHYCARDIAS

If a focus in the ventricular muscle depolarizes with high frequency (causing, in effect, rapidly repeated ventricular extrasystoles), the rhythm is called 'ventricular tachycardia' (Fig. 3.22).

Excitation has to spread by an abnormal path through the ventricular muscle, and the QRS complex is therefore wide and abnormal. Wide and abnormal complexes are seen in all 12 leads of the standard ECG (Fig. 3.23).

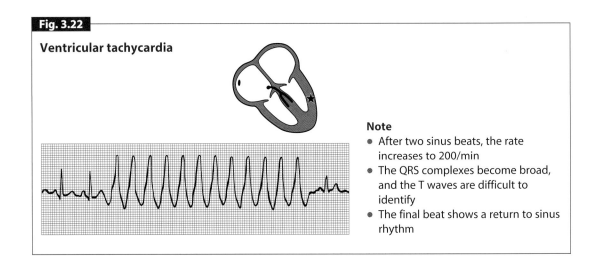

Fig. 3.22

Ventricular tachycardia

Note
- After two sinus beats, the rate increases to 200/min
- The QRS complexes become broad, and the T waves are difficult to identify
- The final beat shows a return to sinus rhythm

ECG
IP

For more about broad complex tachycardias, see p. 110

Fig. 3.23

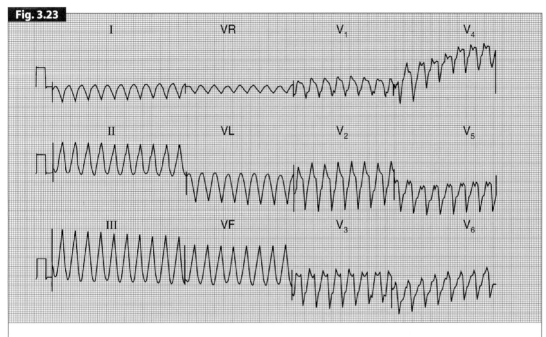

Ventricular tachycardia

Note

- No P waves
- Regular QRS complexes, rate 200/min
- Broad QRS complexes, duration 280 ms, with a very abnormal shape
- No identifiable T waves

ECG
IP

For more about non-ST segment myocardial infarction and ischaemia, see pp. 189–194

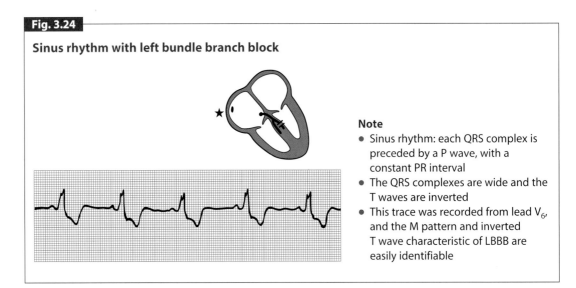

Fig. 3.24

Sinus rhythm with left bundle branch block

Note
- Sinus rhythm: each QRS complex is preceded by a P wave, with a constant PR interval
- The QRS complexes are wide and the T waves are inverted
- This trace was recorded from lead V_6, and the M pattern and inverted T wave characteristic of LBBB are easily identifiable

Remember that wide and abnormal complexes are also seen with bundle branch block (Fig. 3.24).

HOW TO DISTINGUISH BETWEEN VENTRICULAR TACHYCARDIA AND SUPRAVENTRICULAR TACHYCARDIA WITH BUNDLE BRANCH BLOCK

It is essential to remember that the patient's clinical state – whether good or bad – does not help to differentiate between the two possible causes of a tachycardia with broad QRS complexes. If a patient with an acute myocardial infarction has a broad complex tachycardia it will almost always be a ventricular tachycardia. However, a patient with episodes of broad complex tachycardia but without an infarction could be having either a ventricular tachycardia or a supraventricular tachycardia with bundle branch block. Under such circumstances the following points may be helpful:

1. Finding P waves and seeing how they relate to the QRS complexes is always the key to identifying arrhythmias. Always look carefully at a full 12-lead ECG.
2. If possible, compare the QRS complex during the tachycardia with that during sinus rhythm. If the patient has bundle branch block when in sinus rhythm, the QRS complex during the tachycardia will have the same shape as during normal rhythm.
3. If the QRS complex is wider than four small squares (160 ms), the rhythm will probably be ventricular in origin.
4. Left axis deviation during the tachycardia usually indicates a ventricular origin, as does any change of axis compared with a record taken during sinus rhythm.
5. If during the tachycardia the QRS complex is very irregular, the rhythm is probably atrial fibrillation with bundle branch block (see below).

FIBRILLATION

All the arrhythmias discussed so far have involved the synchronous contraction of all the muscle fibres of the atria or of the ventricles, albeit at abnormal speeds. When individual muscle fibres contract independently they are said to be 'fibrillating'. Fibrillation can occur in the atrial or ventricular muscle.

ATRIAL FIBRILLATION

When the atrial muscle fibres contract independently there are no P waves on the ECG, only an irregular line (Fig. 3.25). At times there may be flutter-like waves for 2–3 s. The AV node is continuously bombarded with depolarization waves of varying strength, and depolarization spreads at irregular intervals down the bundle of His. The AV node conducts in an 'all or none' fashion, so that the depolarization waves passing into the His bundle are of constant intensity. However, these waves are irregular and the ventricles therefore contract irregularly.

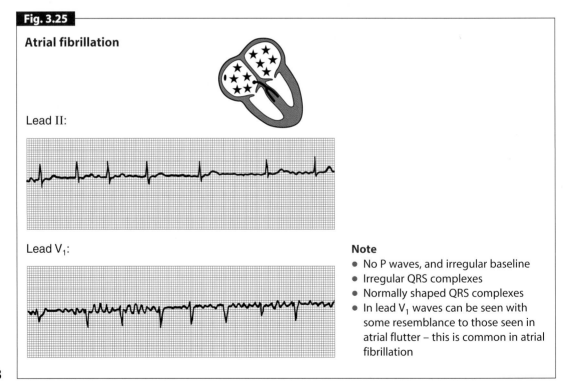

Fig. 3.25

Atrial fibrillation

Lead II:

Lead V₁:

Note
- No P waves, and irregular baseline
- Irregular QRS complexes
- Normally shaped QRS complexes
- In lead V₁ waves can be seen with some resemblance to those seen in atrial flutter – this is common in atrial fibrillation

Because conduction into and through the ventricles is by the normal route, each QRS complex is of normal shape.

In a 12-lead record, fibrillation waves can often be seen much better in some leads than in others (Fig. 3.26).

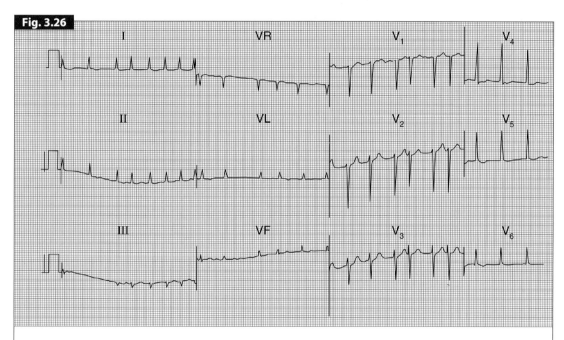

Fig. 3.26

Atrial fibrillation

Note
- No P waves
- Irregular baseline
- Irregular QRS complexes, rate varying between 75 and 190/min
- Narrow QRS complexes of normal shape
- Depressed ST segments in leads V_5–V_6 (digoxin effect – see p. 114)
- Normal T waves

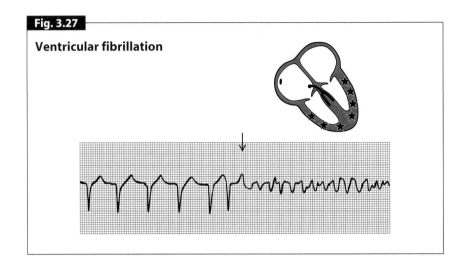

Fig. 3.27

Ventricular fibrillation

VENTRICULAR FIBRILLATION

When the ventricular muscle fibres contract independently, no QRS complex can be identified and the ECG is totally disorganized (Fig. 3.27).

As the patient will usually have lost consciousness by the time you have realized that the change in the ECG pattern is not just due to a loose connection, the diagnosis is easy.

THE WOLFF–PARKINSON–WHITE (WPW) SYNDROME

The only normal electrical connection between the atria and ventricles is the His bundle. Some people, however, have an extra or 'accessory' conducting bundle. Accessory bundles form a direct connection between atrium and ventricle, usually on the left side of the heart, and in the accessory bundle there is no AV node to delay conduction. A depolarization wave therefore reaches the ventricle early and

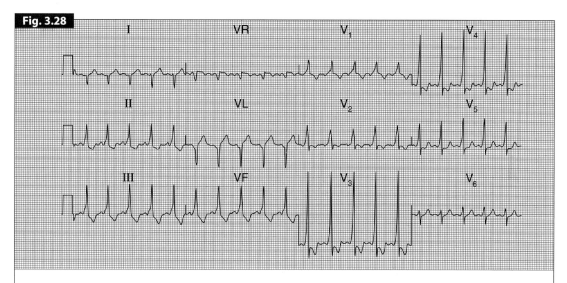

Fig. 3.28

The Wolff–Parkinson–White syndrome

Note
- Sinus rhythm
- Right axis deviation
- Short PR interval
- Slurred upstroke of the QRS complex, best seen in leads V_3 and V_4. Widened QRS complex due to this 'delta' wave
- Dominant R wave in lead V_1

'pre-excitation' occurs. The PR interval is short and the QRS complex shows an early slurred upstroke called a 'delta wave' (Fig. 3.28). The second part of the QRS complex is normal, as conduction through the His bundle catches up with the pre-excitation.

The only clinical importance of this anatomical abnormality is that it can cause paroxysmal tachycardia. Depolarization can spread down the His bundle and back up the accessory pathway, and so reactivate the

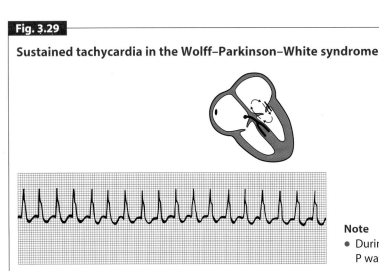

Fig. 3.29

Sustained tachycardia in the Wolff–Parkinson–White syndrome

Note
- During re-entry tachycardia, no P waves can be seen

atrium. A 're-entry' circuit is thus set up, and a sustained tachycardia occurs (Fig. 3.29).

THE ORIGINS OF TACHYCARDIAS

We have considered the tachycardias up to now as if all were due to an increased spontaneous frequency of depolarization of some part of the heart. While such an 'enhanced automaticity' certainly accounts for some tachycardias, others are due to re-entry circuits within the heart muscle. The tachycardias that we have described as 'junctional' are usually due to re-entry circuits around the AV node, and are therefore more properly called 'atrioventricular nodal re-entry (AVNRE) tachycardias'. It is not possible to distinguish enhanced automaticity from re-entry tachycardia on standard ECGs, but fortunately this differentiation has no practical importance.

WHAT TO DO

Accurate interpretation of the ECG is an essential part of arrhythmia management. Although this book is not intended to discuss therapy in detail, it seems appropriate to outline some simple approaches to patient management that logically follow interpretation of an ECG recording:

1. For fast or slow sinus rhythm, treat the underlying cause, not the rhythm itself.
2. Extrasystoles rarely need treatment.
3. In patients with acute heart failure or low blood pressure due to a tachycardia, DC cardioversion should be considered early on.
4. Patients with any bradycardia that is affecting the circulation can be treated with atropine, but if this is ineffective they will need temporary or permanent pacing (Fig. 3.30).
5. The first treatment for any abnormal tachycardia is carotid sinus pressure. This should be performed with the ECG running, and may help make the diagnosis:
   — Sinus tachycardia: carotid sinus pressure causes temporary slowing of the heart rate.

Fig. 3.30

Pacemaker

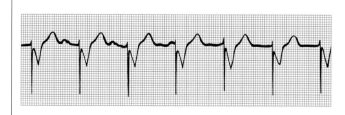

Note
- Occasional P waves are visible, but are not related to the QRS complexes
- The QRS complexes are preceded by a brief spike, representing the pacemaker stimulus
- The QRS complexes are broad, because pacemakers stimulate the right ventricle and cause 'ventricular' beats

— Atrial and junctional tachycardia: carotid sinus pressure may terminate the arrhythmia or may have no effect.
— Atrial flutter: carotid sinus pressure usually causes a temporary increase in block (e.g. from 2:1 to 3:1).
— Atrial fibrillation and ventricular tachycardia: carotid sinus pressure has no effect.

6. Narrow complex tachycardias should be treated initially with adenosine.
7. Wide complex tachycardias should be treated initially with lignocaine.

THINGS TO REMEMBER

1. Most parts of the heart are capable of spontaneous depolarization.
2. Abnormal rhythms can arise in the atrial muscle, the region around the AV node (the junctional region) and in the ventricular muscle.
3. Escape rhythms are slow and are protective.
4. Occasional early depolarization of any part of the heart causes an extrasystole.
5. Frequent depolarization of any part of the heart causes a tachycardia.
6. Asynchronous contraction of muscle fibres in the atria or ventricles is called fibrillation.
7. Apart from the rate, the ECG pattern of an escape rhythm, an extrasystole and a tachycardia arising in any one part of the heart are the same.
8. All supraventricular rhythms have normal QRS complexes provided there is no bundle branch block.
9. Ventricular rhythms cause wide and abnormal QRS complexes, and abnormal T waves.

Recognizing ECG abnormalities is to a large extent like recognizing an elephant – once seen, never forgotten. However, in cases of difficulty it is helpful to ask the following questions, referring to Table 3.1:

1. Is the abnormality occasional or sustained?
2. Are there any P waves?
3. Are there as many QRS complexes as P waves?
4. Are the ventricles contracting regularly or irregularly?
5. Is the QRS complex of normal shape?
6. What is the ventricular rate?

ECG
IP

For more about
tachycardias, see
pp. 99–130

Table 3.1 Recognizing ECG abnormalities

Abnormality	P wave	P:QRS ratio	QRS regularity	QRS shape	QRS rate	Rhythm
Occasional (i.e. extrasystoles)				Normal		Supraventricular
				Abnormal		Ventricular
Sustained	Present	P:QRS = 1:1	Regular	Normal	Normal	Sinus rhythm
					≥ 150/min	Atrial tachycardia
			Slightly irregular	Normal	Normal	Sinus arrhythmia
					Slow	Atrial escape
		More P waves than QRS complexes	Regular	Normal	Fast	Atrial tachycardia with block
					Slow	Second degree heart block
				Abnormal	Slow	Complete heart block
	Absent		Regular	Normal	Fast	Nodal tachycardia
					Slow	Nodal escape
				Abnormal	Fast	Nodal tachycardia with bundle branch block or ventricular tachycardia
			Slightly irregular	Abnormal	Fast	Ventricular tachycardia
			Very irregular	Normal	Any speed	Atrial fibrillation
				Abnormal	Any speed	Atrial fibrillation and bundle branch block
		QRS complexes absent				Ventricular fibrillation or standstill

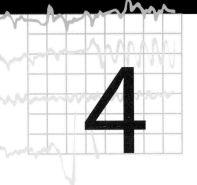

4

Abnormalities of P waves, QRS complexes and T waves

When interpreting an ECG, identify the rhythm first. Then ask the following questions – always in the same sequence:

1. Are there any abnormalities of the P wave?
2. What is the direction of the cardiac axis? (Look at the QRS complex in leads I, II, III – and at Ch. 1 if necessary.)
3. Is the QRS complex of normal duration?
4. Are there any abnormalities in the QRS complex – particularly, are there any abnormal Q waves?

5. Is the ST segment raised or depressed?
6. Is the T wave normal?

Remember:

1. The P wave can only be normal, unusually tall, or unusually broad.
2. The QRS complex can only have three abnormalities – it can be too broad, too tall, and it may contain an abnormal Q wave.
3. The ST segment can only be normal, elevated or depressed.
4. The T wave can only be the right way up or the wrong way up.

ABNORMALITIES OF THE P WAVE

Apart from alterations of the shape of the P wave associated with rhythm changes, there are only two important abnormalities:

1. Anything that causes the right atrium to become hypertrophied (such as tricuspid valve stenosis or pulmonary hypertension) causes the P wave to become peaked (Fig. 4.1).
2. Left atrial hypertrophy (usually due to mitral stenosis) causes a broad and bifid P wave (Fig. 4.2).

Fig. 4.1

Right atrial hypertrophy

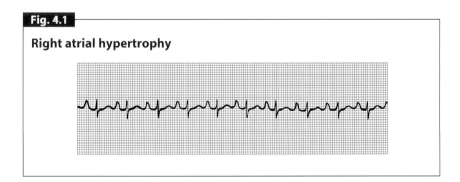

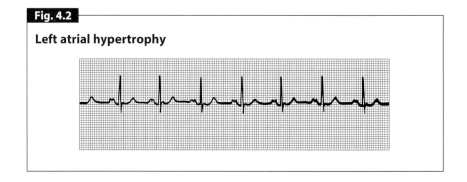

Fig. 4.2

Left atrial hypertrophy

ABNORMALITIES OF THE QRS COMPLEX

The normal QRS complex has four characteristics:

1. Its duration is no greater than 120 ms (three small squares).
2. In a right ventricular lead (V_1), the S wave is greater than the R wave.
3. In a left ventricular lead (V_5 or V_6), the height of the R wave is less than 25 mm.
4. Left ventricular leads may show Q waves due to septal depolarization, but these are less than 1 mm across and less than 2 mm deep.

ABNORMALITIES OF THE WIDTH OF THE QRS COMPLEX

QRS complexes are abnormally wide in the presence of bundle branch block (see Ch. 2), or when depolarization is initiated by a focus in the ventricular muscle causing ventricular escape beats, extrasystoles or tachycardia (see Ch. 3). In each case, the increased width indicates that depolarization has spread through the ventricles by an abnormal and therefore slow pathway.

INCREASED HEIGHT OF THE QRS COMPLEX

An increase of muscle mass in either ventricle will lead to increased electrical activity, and to an increase in the height of the QRS complex.

Right ventricular hypertrophy

Right ventricular hypertrophy is best seen in the right ventricular leads (especially V_1). Since the left ventricle does not have its usual dominant effect on the QRS shape, the complex in lead V_1 becomes upright (i.e. the height of the R wave exceeds the depth of the S wave) – this is nearly always abnormal (Fig. 4.3). There will also be a deep S wave in lead V_6.

Fig. 4.3

The QRS complex in right ventricular hypertrophy

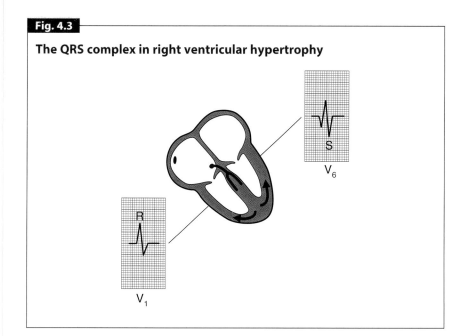

1. Peaked P waves.
2. Right axis deviation (S waves in lead I).
3. Tall R waves in lead V_1.
4. Right bundle branch block.
5. Inverted T waves in lead V_1 (normal), spreading across to lead V_2 or V_3.
6. A shift of transition point to the left, so that the R wave equals the S wave in lead V_5 or V_6 rather than in lead V_3 or V_4 (clockwise rotation). A deep S wave will persist in lead V_6.
7. Curiously, a 'Q' wave in lead III resembling an inferior infarction (see below).

However, do not hesitate to treat the patient if the clinical picture suggests pulmonary embolism but the ECG does not show the classical pattern of right ventricular hypertrophy. If in doubt, treat the patient with an anticoagulant.

Left ventricular hypertrophy

Left ventricular hypertrophy causes a tall R wave (greater than 25 mm) in lead V_5 or V_6 and a deep S wave in lead V_1 or V_2 (Fig. 4.6) – but in practice such 'voltage' changes alone are unhelpful in diagnosing left ventricular enlargement. With significant hypertrophy, there are also inverted T waves in leads I, VL, V_5 and V_6, and sometimes V_4, and there may be left axis deviation. It is difficult to diagnose minor degrees of left ventricular hypertrophy from the ECG.

THE ORIGIN OF Q WAVES

Small (septal) 'Q' waves in the left ventricular leads result from depolarization of the septum from left to right (see Ch. 1). However, Q waves greater than one small square in width (representing 40 ms), and greater than 2 mm in depth have a quite different significance.

Fig. 4.6

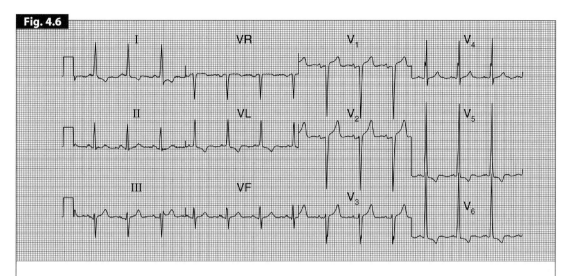

Left ventricular hypertrophy

Note

- Sinus rhythm
- Normal axis
- Tall R waves in leads V_5–V_6, and deep S waves in leads V_1–V_2 (R wave in lead V_5, 40 mm)
- Inverted T waves in leads I, VL, V_5–V_6

The ventricles are depolarized from inside outwards (Fig. 4.7). Therefore, an electrode placed in the cavity of a ventricle would record only a Q wave, because all the depolarization waves would be moving away from it. If a myocardial infarction causes complete death of muscle from the inside surface to the outside surface of the heart, an electrical 'window' is created, and an electrode looking at the heart over that window will record a cavity potential – that is, a Q wave.

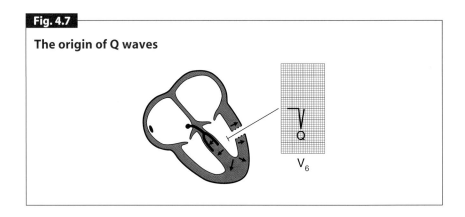

Fig. 4.7

The origin of Q waves

Q waves greater than one small square in width and at least 2 mm deep therefore indicate a myocardial infarction, and the leads in which the Q wave appears give some indication of the part of the heart that has been damaged. Thus, infarction of the anterior wall of the left ventricle causes a Q wave in the leads looking at the heart from the front – V_2–V_4 or V_5 (Fig. 4.8) (see Ch. 1 and Fig. 4.15).

If the infarction involves both the anterior and lateral surfaces of the heart, a Q wave will be present in leads V_3 and V_4 and in the leads that look at the lateral surface – I, VL and V_5–V_6 (Fig. 4.9).

Infarctions of the inferior surface of the heart cause Q waves in the leads looking at the heart from below – III and VF (Figs 4.8 and 4.10).

When the posterior wall of the left ventricle is infarcted, a different pattern is seen (Fig. 4.11). The right ventricle occupies the front of the heart anatomically, and normally depolarization of the right ventricle (moving towards the recording electrode V_1) is overshadowed by depolarization of the left ventricle (moving away from V_1). The result is a dominant S wave in lead V_1. With infarction of the posterior wall of the left ventricle, depolarization of the right ventricle is less opposed by left ventricular forces, and so becomes more obvious and a dominant R wave develops in lead V_1. The appearance of the ECG is similar to

Fig. 4.8

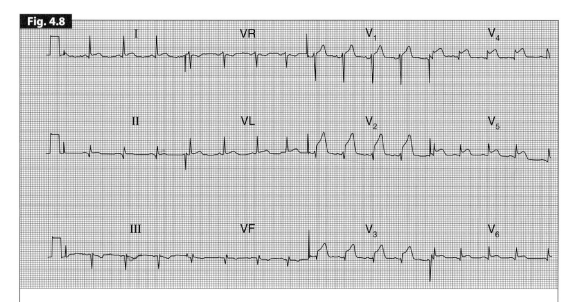

Acute anterior myocardial infarction, and probable old inferior infarction

Note
- Sinus rhythm with a normal axis
- Small Q waves in leads II, III, VF – associated with flat ST segments and inverted T waves, indicate old inferior infarction
- Small Q waves in leads V_3–V_4 – associated with raised ST segments, indicate acute anterior infarction
- See also Fig. 4.15

that of right ventricular hypertrophy, though the other changes of right ventricular hypertrophy (see above) do not appear.

The presence of a Q wave does not give any indication of the age of an infarction, because once a Q wave has developed it is usually permanent.

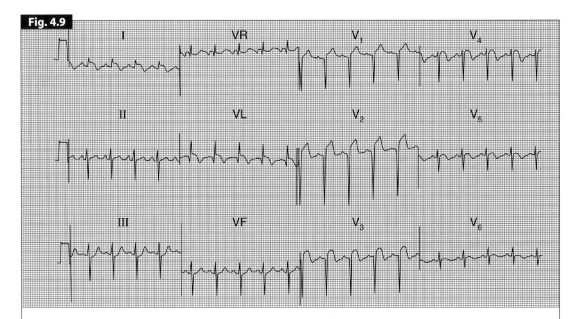

Fig. 4.9

Acute anterolateral myocardial infarction and left anterior hemiblock

Note
- Sinus rhythm
- Left axis deviation (dominant S waves in leads II and III)
- Q waves in leads VL, V_2–V_3
- Raised ST segments in leads I, VL, V_2–V_5

ECG
IP

For more about
myocardial infarction,
see pp. 165–189

Fig. 4.10

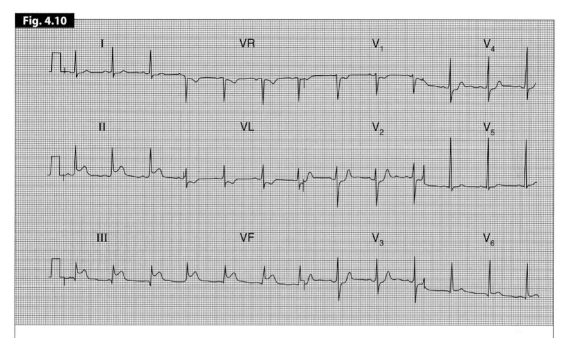

Acute inferior infarction; lateral ischaemia

Note
- Sinus rhythm
- Normal axis
- Q waves in leads III, VF
- Normal QRS complexes
- Raised ST segments in leads II, III, VF
- Inverted T waves in lead VL (abnormal) and in lead V_1 (normal)

damaged – anterior damage shows in the V leads, and inferior damage in leads III and VF (see Figs 4.8 and 4.10). Pericarditis is not usually a localized affair, and so it causes ST elevation in most leads.

Horizontal depression of the ST segment, associated with an upright T wave, is usually a sign of ischaemia as opposed to infarction. When the ECG at rest is normal, ST segment depression may appear during exercise, particularly when effort induces angina (Fig. 4.14).

Downward-sloping, as opposed to horizontally depressed, ST segments are usually due to treatment with digoxin (described later).

Fig. 4.14

Exercise-induced ischaemic changes

Rest:

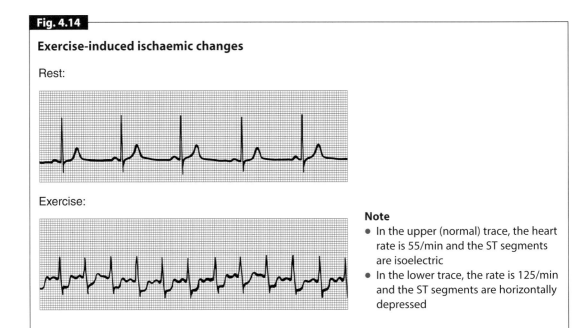

Exercise:

Note
- In the upper (normal) trace, the heart rate is 55/min and the ST segments are isoelectric
- In the lower trace, the rate is 125/min and the ST segments are horizontally depressed

ABNORMALITIES OF THE T WAVE

INVERSION OF THE T WAVE

The T wave is normally inverted in leads VR and V_1, sometimes in leads III and V_2, and also in lead V_3 in some black people.

T wave inversion is seen in the following circumstances:

1. normality
2. ischaemia
3. ventricular hypertrophy
4. bundle branch block
5. digoxin treatment.

Leads adjacent to those showing inverted T waves sometimes show 'biphasic' T waves – initially upright and then inverted.

MYOCARDIAL INFARCTION

After a myocardial infarction, the first abnormality seen on the ECG is elevation of the ST segment (Fig. 4.15). Subsequently Q waves appear, and the T waves become inverted. The ST segment returns to the baseline, the whole process taking a variable time but usually within the range 24–48 h. T wave inversion is often permanent. Infarctions causing this pattern of ECG changes are called 'ST segment elevation myocardial infarctions' (STEMIs) (see p. 130).

If an infarction is not full thickness and so does not cause an electrical window, there will be T wave inversion but no Q waves (Fig. 4.16). Infarctions with this pattern of ECG change are called 'non-ST segment elevation myocardial infarctions' (NSTEMIs). The older term for the same pattern was 'non-Q wave infarction' or 'subendocardial infarction'.

Fig. 4.15

Development of inferior infarction

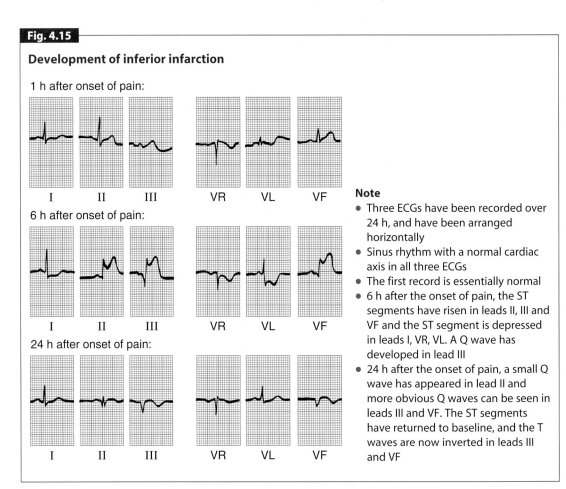

1 h after onset of pain:

I   II   III   VR   VL   VF

6 h after onset of pain:

I   II   III   VR   VL   VF

24 h after onset of pain:

I   II   III   VR   VL   VF

Note

- Three ECGs have been recorded over 24 h, and have been arranged horizontally
- Sinus rhythm with a normal cardiac axis in all three ECGs
- The first record is essentially normal
- 6 h after the onset of pain, the ST segments have risen in leads II, III and VF and the ST segment is depressed in leads I, VR, VL. A Q wave has developed in lead III
- 24 h after the onset of pain, a small Q wave has appeared in lead II and more obvious Q waves can be seen in leads III and VF. The ST segments have returned to baseline, and the T waves are now inverted in leads III and VF

Fig. 4.16

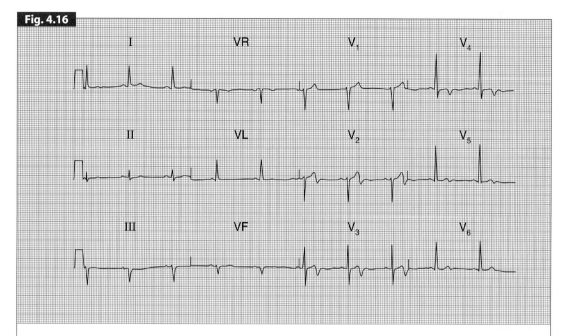

Anterior non-ST segment elevation myocardial infarction

Note
- Sinus rhythm
- Normal axis
- Normal QRS complexes
- Inverted T waves in leads V_3–V_4
- Biphasic T waves in leads V_2 and V_5

VENTRICULAR HYPERTROPHY

Left ventricular hypertrophy causes inverted T waves in leads looking at the left ventricle (I, II, VL, V_5–V_6) (see Fig. 4.6). Right ventricular hypertrophy causes T wave inversion in the leads looking at the right ventricle (T wave inversion is normal in lead V_1, but in white adults is abnormal in leads V_2 or V_3) (see Fig. 4.4).

BUNDLE BRANCH BLOCK

The abnormal path of depolarization in bundle branch block is usually associated with an abnormal path of repolarization. Therefore, inverted T waves associated with QRS complexes which have a duration of 160 ms or more have no significance in themselves (see Figs 2.15 and 2.16).

DIGOXIN

The administration of digoxin causes T wave inversion, characteristically with sloping depression of the ST segment (Fig. 4.17). It is helpful to record an ECG before giving digoxin, to save later confusion about the significance of T wave changes.

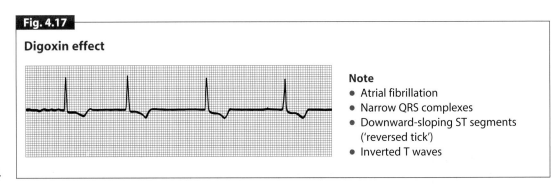

Fig. 4.17

Digoxin effect

Note
- Atrial fibrillation
- Narrow QRS complexes
- Downward-sloping ST segments ('reversed tick')
- Inverted T waves

OTHER ABNORMALITIES OF THE ST SEGMENT AND THE T WAVE

ELECTROLYTE ABNORMALITIES

Abnormalities of the plasma levels of potassium, calcium and magnesium affect the ECG, though changes in the plasma sodium level do not. The T wave and QT interval (measured from the onset of the QRS complex to the end of the T wave) are most commonly affected.

A low potassium level causes T wave flattening and the appearance of a hump on the end of the T wave called a 'U' wave. A high potassium level causes peaked T waves with the disappearance of the ST segment. The QRS complex may be widened. The effects of abnormal magnesium levels are similar.

A low plasma calcium level causes prolongation of the QT interval, and a high plasma calcium level shortens it.

NONSPECIFIC CHANGES

Minor degrees of ST segment and T wave abnormalities (T wave flattening, etc.) are usually of no great significance, and are best reported as 'nonspecific ST–T changes'.

THINGS TO REMEMBER

1. Tall P waves result from right atrial hypertrophy, and broad P waves from left atrial hypertrophy.
2. Broadening of the QRS complex indicates abnormal intraventricular conduction: it is seen in bundle branch block and in complexes originating in the ventricular muscle.
3. Increased height of the QRS complex indicates ventricular hypertrophy. Right ventricular hypertrophy is seen in lead V_1, and left ventricular hypertrophy is seen in leads V_5–V_6.

4. Q waves greater than 1 mm across and 2 mm deep indicate myocardial infarction.
5. ST segment elevation indicates acute myocardial infarction or pericarditis.
6. ST segment depression and T wave inversion may be due to ischaemia, ventricular hypertrophy, abnormal intraventricular conduction, or digoxin.
7. T wave inversion is normal in leads III, VR and V_1. T wave inversion is associated with bundle branch block, ischaemia, and ventricular hypertrophy.
8. T wave flattening or peaking with an unusually long or short QT interval may be due to electrolyte abnormalities, but many minor ST–T changes are nonspecific.

And finally, remember:

- The ECG is easy to understand.
- Most abnormalities of the ECG are amenable to reason.

ECG
IP

For more about the effect of electrolyte abnormalities, see p. 266

How to use the ECG

The ECG must be used as an addition to, and not as a substitute for, proper history-taking and proper physical examination. If the ECG is used without thinking carefully about the patient from whom it was recorded, disastrous diagnosis and treatment may occur. When you have recorded an ECG, consider how it fits in with the patient's symptoms and signs, and then think about conditions that might be responsible for any abnormalities detected, and about possible treatment.

It is important to ask whether the patient had any symptoms at the time the ECG was recorded. This is particularly important in the case of patients who complain of palpitations (which can be defined as an awareness of the heartbeat): if the patient was asymptomatic at the time there may nevertheless be abnormalities, but a confident diagnosis can only be made if the ECG record actually corresponds with the symptoms. Similarly with chest pain: the ECG will only be totally reliable if the patient has pain at the time of the recording.

It is essential always to bear in mind the limits of normality of the ECG: there are many variations of 'normal' which resemble important abnormalities.

Every ECG must be related to a patient, so this chapter considers the use of the ECG in the main patient groups in whom records are made:

- Healthy subjects in whom the ECG is used as some sort of health check.
- Patients with palpitations (in whom the ECG is the only certain way of making a diagnosis).
- Patients with chest pain.
- Patients with breathlessness.

This covers the important conditions in which an ECG is helpful. For more detailed consideration, including the situations in which 'normal' and 'abnormal' ECGs resemble each other, see the companion volume, *The ECG in Practice*.

THE ECG IN HEALTHY PATIENTS

An ECG may be recorded in the absence of symptoms from patients in specific occupations, such as airline pilots and athletes. Its function in these cases is to detect conditions such as hypertrophic cardiomyopathy which might lead to sudden death, for example due to strenuous activity. Most 'healthy' patients asking for ECGs are undergoing routine health checks, but it is important to remember that these patients may actually have symptoms which they have not declared. A normal ECG never disproves the presence of heart disease, though it may make it less likely; conversely, a lot of apparent abnormalities in the ECG may actually be normal variants. Sometimes, however, true and significant abnormalities are detected during routine checks.

THE CARDIAC RHYTHM

The only totally normal rhythm is sinus rhythm, but there is a wide range of normality in the sinus rate and there are no precise limits outside which the terms 'sinus tachycardia' or 'sinus bradycardia' can be used. Figure 5.1 shows the ECG recorded from a patient with a fast heart rate; no abnormalities were found on examination.

If the heart rate seems surprisingly fast or slow, consider the possible causes (Box 5.1).

Fig. 5.1

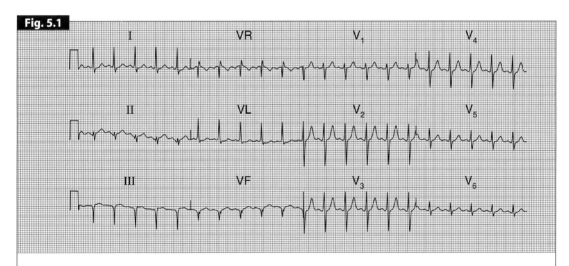

Sinus tachycardia: normal ECG

Note
- Heart rate 128/min
- Sinus rhythm – one P wave per QRS complex
- Left axis deviation – dominant S waves in leads II and III
- Normal QRS complexes and T waves

Box 5.1 Causes of fast or slow heart rate

Sinus tachycardia	Sinus bradycardia
• Exercise	• Physical fitness
• Pain	• Vasovagal attacks
• Fright	• Hypothermia
• Obesity	• Hypothyroidism
• Pregnancy	
• Anaemia	
• Thyrotoxicosis	
• CO_2 retention	

CONDUCTION

Subjects with normal hearts may show first degree heart block, and sometimes right bundle branch block (RBBB), though the latter may be an indication for further investigation by echocardiography. RBBB with a QRS complex duration of less than 120 ms (three small squares) can be accepted as a normal variant (Fig. 5.2).

Left bundle branch block, even as a finding in an apparently healthy subject, is always abnormal.

The possible causes of bundle branch block are summarized in Box 5.2.

THE QRS COMPLEX

Small Q waves may be normal. The septum is depolarized from left to right, so the leads looking at the left ventricle (I, II, VL, V_5–V_6) can show a 'septal' Q wave which is perfectly normal and does not indicate a myocardial infarction. There can also be a normal Q wave in lead III. Septal Q waves are usually less than 1 mm wide and usually less than 2 mm deep (Fig. 5.3), although this is not always the case.

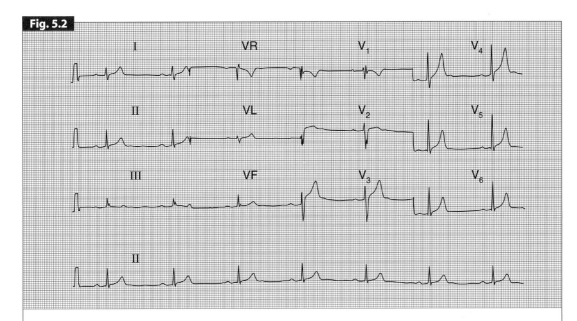

Fig. 5.2

First degree block and partial right bundle branch block

Note
- Sinus rhythm
- PR interval 256 ms – first degree block
- Normal axis
- Normal QRS complex duration – 110 ms
- RSR[1] complex in leads V_1–V_2 – partial RBBB

Box 5.2 Causes of bundle branch block

Right bundle branch block	Left bundle branch block
- Normal heart	- Ischaemia
- Atrial septal defect or other congenital disease	- Aortic stenosis
	- Hypertension
- Pulmonary embolism	- Cardiomyopathy

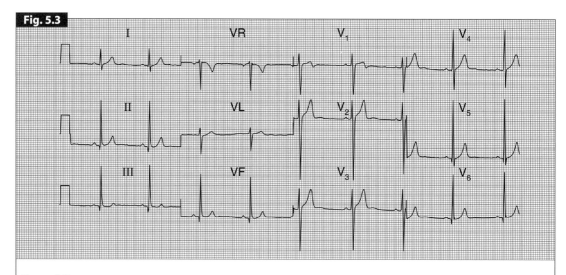

Fig. 5.3

Septal Q waves

Note
- Sinus rhythm
- Normal PR interval
- Normal axis
- QRS complexes show narrow Q waves in leads II, III, VF, V_5–V_6: septal Q waves
- Normal ST segments and T waves

A tall R wave in lead V_1 is a sign of right ventricular hypertrophy, but it can also occur in normal hearts. The height of the QRS complex in the left chest leads should not exceed 25 mm, and the combined maximum height of the R wave in lead V_5 or V_6 and the maximum depth of the S wave in lead V_1 should not exceed 35 mm. Beyond these limits, the 'voltage criteria' for left ventricular hypertrophy are said to exist (Fig. 5.4). In fact this is a very poor marker for left ventricular hypertrophy, and the pattern is often seen in fit young people, particularly athletes.

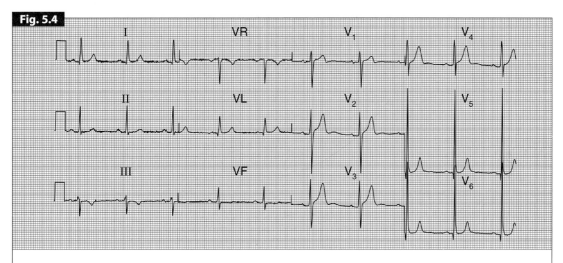

Fig. 5.4

Left ventricular hypertrophy (on voltage criteria only)

Note

- Sinus rhythm
- Normal PR interval
- Normal axis
- QRS complex: R wave = 45 mm in lead V_5; S wave = 15 mm in lead V_1
- Normal T waves
- Small normal U waves
- Check the calibration – correct at 1 mV = 1 cm

THE ST SEGMENT

A raised ST segment is characteristic of myocardial infarction and (less commonly) of pericarditis, but it can also be a normal variant when it follows an S wave (Fig. 5.5). This is important, because unless the pattern is recognized, a false diagnosis of myocardial infarction may be made and the patient may inappropriately be given thrombolytic treatment. A raised ST segment beginning after an S wave is called 'high take-off', and is perfectly normal.

123

Palpitations may be associated with extrasystoles, paroxysmal tachycardia or simply an awareness of sinus rhythm.

Extrasystoles can be identified from a story of sudden single beats – though of course what the patient is noticing is the normal sinus beat that follows the extrasystole, because of the increased stroke output follows the extrasystole.

In paroxysmal tachycardia the attack begins suddenly, and if a story is obtained of a sudden cessation of the tachycardia the diagnosis is virtually certain. If the palpitations are associated with chest pain (suggesting angina), dizziness (cerebral hypoperfusion) or breathlessness (heart failure), then it is likely that the patient is describing paroxysmal tachycardia.

In sinus tachycardia, the heart speeds up and slows down, and attacks usually have an identifiable cause such as anxiety.

When the patient is asymptomatic the ECG can still be useful – it may show evidence of ischaemia or cardiomyopathy, which could suggest that the patient is prone to arrhythmias, or there may be evidence of pre-excitation (see p. 91)

Recording an ECG when the patient has symptoms is the only certain way of identifying an arrhythmia. In a patient with an irregular pulse, the ECG will differentiate between extrasystoles and atrial fibrillation (see pp. 73 and 88), and in a patient with a rapid pulse it will distinguish between supraventricular and ventricular tachycardia (see pp. 86–87). An ECG should always be recorded when an attempt is made to terminate a tachycardia by carotid sinus pressure.

THE ECG IN PATIENTS WITH CHEST PAIN

As with palpitations, a carefully-taken history is more important than the ECG. The main problem is usually differentiating between pain due to cardiac ischaemia and the nonspecific chest pain that is common in middle-aged men and which, for no very good reason, is often labelled musculoskeletal.

Ischaemic pain is typically central and may radiate to the arms or back; when there is radiation to the jaw or teeth the diagnosis is virtually certain. Pain due to angina is above all predictable, either at a fairly constant level of exercise or in response to emotional stress. Pain due to myocardial infarction is usually – but not always – severe, and is associated with sweating or vomiting.

But there are many other causes of chest pain, most of which can mimic cardiac ischaemia (see Box 5.3).

The important thing to remember is that in a patient with cardiac ischaemia the ECG can be normal, and then it is better to believe the history than the ECG. If pain occurs during exercise then an exercise test may help; if the pain sounds like an infarction then the patient should be admitted to hospital for sufficient time for changes to occur in the ECG if they are going to do so, and for other markers of infarction such as the plasma troponin level to be measured.

Box 5.3 Causes of chest pain

Acute chest pain	Intermittent chest pain
• Myocardial infarction	• Angina
• Pulmonary embolism	• Oesophageal pain
• Pneumothorax and other pleuritic disease	• Muscular pain
• Pericarditis	• Nonspecific pain
• Aortic dissection	

For more about the
ECG in patients
with chest pain, see
Chapter 3

THE ECG IN CARDIAC ISCHAEMIA

Remember – the ECG may be normal.

In a patient with chest pain that could be due to angina, the ECG may show evidence of an old infarction, which would tend to confirm that the patient might indeed have angina (Fig. 5.7).

Fig. 5.7

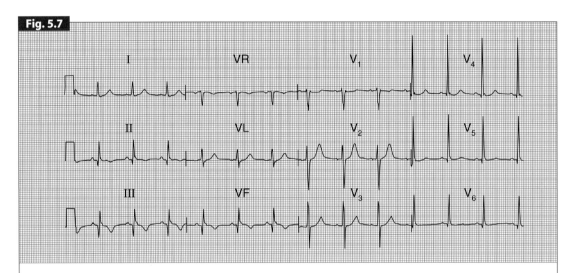

Old inferior myocardial infarction

Note
- Sinus rhythm
- Normal PR interval
- Normal axis
- Prominent and deep Q waves in leads II, III and VF, indicating an inferior infarction. There are also small Q waves in leads V_5–V_6, but these may be septal
- ST segments normal, with no elevation in the leads showing Q waves
- Inverted T waves in leads II, III and VF

If the patient has pain at the time of the recording, there may be horizontal depression of the ST segments (Fig. 5.8). For a firm diagnosis, the ST segment should be depressed by 2 mm; less depression should be regarded as suspicious but not diagnostic.

If the patient seems to have angina, but the ECG shows left ventricular hypertrophy or left bundle branch block, the possibility of aortic stenosis must be considered.

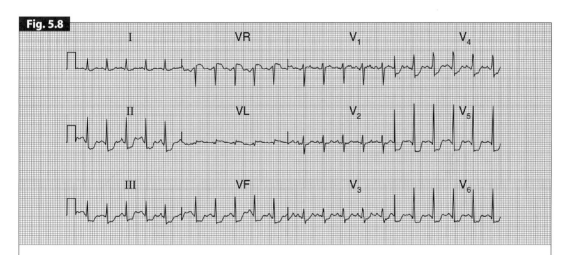

Fig. 5.8

Ischaemic ST segment depression

Note
- ECG recorded during an exercise test; the resting record had been perfectly normal
- Sinus rhythm, rate 130/min
- Normal axis
- Normal QRS complexes
- ST segments depressed horizontally in most leads, but particularly in lead V_5, where the depression is 4 mm

ACUTE CORONARY SYNDROME

The ECG remains of paramount importance in the diagnosis of cardiac ischaemia in general, but its role in the diagnosis of myocardial infarction has to some extent been overtaken by the development of the plasma troponin assay, with its ability to detect small amounts of myocardial necrosis. The plasma troponin level can rise without any accompanying ECG changes if only a very small area of myocardial cell death occurs, although this is rare.

A patient with acute chest pain due to cardiac ischaemia has an acute coronary syndrome. This term includes:

- myocardial infarction
- chest pain with ischaemic ST segment depression but no troponin rise (what used to be called 'unstable angina')
- sudden death due to coronary disease.

In acute coronary syndrome, the ECG may or may not show ST segment elevation. Patients with an acute coronary syndrome whose ECGs do not initially show ST segment elevation and who have a normal plasma troponin level (i.e. patients probably without a myocardial infarction) are said to have 'unstable angina'.

There are two parallel sets of terminology for describing myocardial infarctions, both depending on the ECG appearance:

- STEMI/NSTEMI
- Q wave infarction/non-Q wave infarction.

The elevation (or not) of the ST segment is the criterion underlying the terminology 'STEMI' (ST segment elevation myocardial infarction) and 'NSTEMI' (non-ST segment elevation myocardial infarction). In either case, the patient will usually have a raised plasma troponin level.

In practice, patients with an acute coronary syndrome tend to be described as having a STEMI or an NSTEMI on the basis of the elevation of the ST segments of the ECG, even before the result of the troponin assay is known. This is not technically correct, but early differentiation between a STEMI and an NSTEMI is needed to determine immediate treatment. Patients with a STEMI (Fig. 5.9) need thrombolysis or immediate angioplasty, while patients with an NSTEMI need beta-blockers, heparin and anti-platelet agents. Confusingly, the less specific term 'acute coronary syndrome' is sometimes used to describe NSTEMI but not STEMI.

In parallel with the STEMI/NSTEMI classification, the labels 'Q wave' and 'non-Q wave' infarction are in use, reflecting the appearance

Fig. 5.9

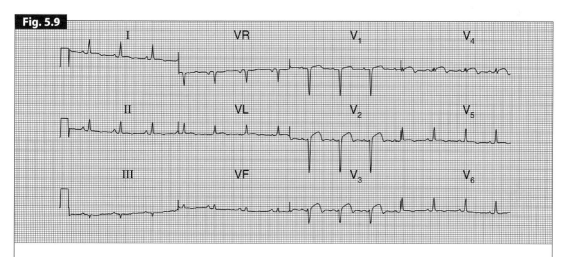

Acute anterior myocardial infarction

Note
- Sinus rhythm
- Normal PR interval
- Normal axis
- QRS complexes mostly normal, but in lead V_3 there is only a very small R wave
- ST segments in leads V_2–V_4 raised by more than 2 mm
- General T wave flattening, with inversion in leads V_5–V_6
- ST segment elevation by more than 2 mm in two adjacent leads (in this case, three adjacent leads, V_2–V_4) indicates that the patient has an acute myocardial infarction, and thrombolysis or immediate angioplasty is indicated

of Q waves on the ECG. The ECG of a patient with a STEMI may show Q waves when the patient is initially seen, but even if not, the ECG of most of these patients will eventually develop Q waves (see Fig. 4.15, p. 111), and then the term 'Q wave infarction' will become appropriate. However, early treatment of a STEMI with thrombolysis or angioplasty may prevent the sequence of ECG changes leading to Q wave formation, and the term 'non-Q wave infarction' will then be appropriate. Patients with an NSTEMI usually have a final ECG that shows T wave changes but no Q waves, so the label 'non-Q wave infarction' can be used.

THE ECG IN PULMONARY EMBOLISM

We have already seen (Ch. 4) that the ECG can show a variety of changes in pulmonary embolism, but it is essential to remember that the most common finding is a normal ECG, probably with sinus tachycardia. A deviation of the cardiac axis to the right, or the appearance of inverted T waves in leads V_2 and V_3 (Fig. 5.10), is more common than the marked changes of right ventricular hypertrophy shown in Figure 4.4.

THE ECG IN PATIENTS WITH BREATHLESSNESS

The causes of breathlessness are summarized in Box 5.4.

It is important to recognize that the ECG cannot diagnose heart failure, though the presence of an abnormal rhythm, or any other evidence of cardiac disease, must raise the possibility that heart failure is present. Patients with valve disease may have evidence of ventricular hypertrophy – left ventricular hypertrophy in the case of aortic stenosis or regurgitation, or of mitral regurgitation, and right ventricular hypertrophy in patients with mitral stenosis (see p. 100).

Any severe lung disease can lead to right ventricular hypertrophy, and the changes in the ECG that we have seen in pulmonary embolism

Fig. 5.10

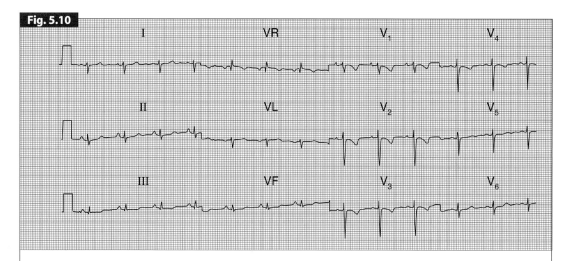

Pulmonary embolism

Note

- Sinus rhythm
- Normal PR interval
- Right axis deviation (dominant S wave in lead I)
- QRS complexes show a dominant S wave in lead V_6. This is sometimes called a 'persistent' S wave, because in the normal ECG there is no S wave in lead V_6
- T wave inversion in leads V_1–V_4. This is maximal in the leads 'looking at' the right ventricle (V_1 and V_2), so it can be assumed that this change is due to a right ventricular problem, and not to septal or left ventricular ischaemia

Box 5.4 Causes of breathlessness

- A lack of physical fitness
- Obesity
- Heart failure
- Lung disease
- Anaemia

ECG
IP

For more about the ECG in patients with breathlessness, see Chapter 4

are therefore not diagnostic. In chronic lung disease, the characteristic change is clockwise rotation, with the right ventricle occupying the front of the chest so that the transition point swings to the left and there is a deep S wave in lead V_6. In other words, the left chest leads never show a fully developed left ventricular complex, and this would only be seen if recordings were made from electrodes placed in the posterior axillary line and round the back of the chest. The main feature of Figure 5.11 is clockwise rotation with no T wave inversion: this is characteristic of chronic lung disease of any sort.

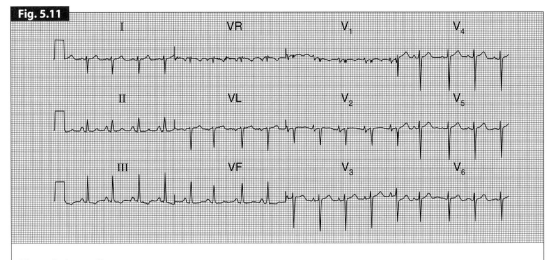

Fig. 5.11

Chronic lung disease

Note

- Sinus rhythm
- Peaked P waves (especially in lead V_2) suggest right atrial hypertrophy
- Right axis deviation (dominant S wave in lead I)
- QRS complexes show a dominant S wave in lead V_6, with no development of a left ventricular complex – this is called 'clockwise rotation'
- Normal ST segments and T waves

134

Reminders

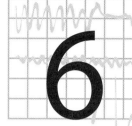

These lists will remind you of the features that will help you recognize the patterns of normality and abnormality in the ECG.

THE NORMAL ECG

LIMITS OF NORMAL DURATIONS
- PR interval: 200 ms (five small squares).
- QRS complex duration: 120 ms (three small squares).
- QT interval: 450 ms.

RHYTHM

- Sinus arrhythmia.
- Supraventricular extrasystoles are always normal.

THE CARDIAC AXIS

- Normal axis: QRS complex predominantly upward in leads I, II and III; still normal if QRS complex is downward in lead III.
- Minor degrees of right and left axis deviation are within the normal range.

QRS COMPLEX

- Small Q waves normal in leads I, VL and V_6 (septal Q waves).
- RSR^1 pattern in lead V_1 normal if the duration is less than 120 ms (partial right bundle branch block).
- R wave smaller than S wave in lead V_1.
- R wave in lead V_6 less than 25 mm.
- R wave in lead V_6 plus S wave in lead V_1 less than 35 mm.

ST SEGMENT

- Should be isoelectric.

T WAVE

- May be inverted in:
  — lead III
  — lead VR
  — lead V_1
  — lead V_2
  — lead V_3, in black people.

WHAT TO LOOK FOR

1. The rhythm.
2. P wave abnormalities:
   — peaked, tall – right atrial hypertrophy
   — notched, broad – left atrial hypertrophy.
3. The cardiac axis:
   — right axis deviation – QRS complex predominantly downward in lead I
   — left axis deviation – QRS complex predominantly downward in leads II and III.
4. The QRS complex:
   — width:
     • if wide, ventricular origin or bundle branch block
   — height:
     • tall R waves in lead V_1 in right ventricular hypertrophy
     • tall R waves in lead V_6 in left ventricular hypertrophy
   — transition point:
     • R and S waves are equal in the chest leads over the interventricular septum (normally lead V_3 or V_4)
     • clockwise rotation indicates chronic lung disease
   — Q waves.
5. The ST segment:
   — raised in acute myocardial infarction and in pericarditis
   — depressed in ischaemia and with digoxin.
6. T waves:
   — peaked in hyperkalaemia
   — flat and prolonged in hypokalaemia
   — inverted:
     • normal in some leads
     • ischaemia
     • infarction
     • left or right ventricular hypertrophy

137

- may be inverted in leads V_1–V_3 in pulmonary embolism
- bundle branch block.

7. U waves:
  — can be normal
  — hypokalaemia.

CONDUCTION PROBLEMS

FIRST DEGREE BLOCK

- One P wave per QRS complex.
- PR interval greater than 200 ms.

SECOND DEGREE BLOCK

- Mobitz type 2: occasional nonconducted beats.
- Wenckebach: progressive lengthening of the PR interval, then nonconducted P wave, followed by repetition of the cycle.
- 2:1 (or 3:1) block: two (or three) P waves per QRS complex, with normal P wave rate.

THIRD DEGREE (COMPLETE) BLOCK

- No relationship between P waves and QRS complexes.
- Usually, wide QRS complexes.
- Usual QRS complex rate less than 50/min.
- Sometimes narrow QRS complexes, rate 50–60/min.

RIGHT BUNDLE BRANCH BLOCK

- QRS complex duration greater than 120 ms.
- RSR^1 pattern.
- Usually, dominant R^1 wave in lead V_1.
- Inverted T waves in lead V_1, and sometimes in leads V_2–V_3.
- Deep and wide S waves in lead V_6.

LEFT ANTERIOR HEMIBLOCK

- Marked left axis deviation – deep S waves in leads II and III, usually with a slightly wide QRS complex.

LEFT BUNDLE BRANCH BLOCK

- QRS complex duration greater than 120 ms.
- M pattern in lead V_6, and sometimes in leads V_4–V_5.
- No septal Q waves.
- Inverted T waves in leads I, VL, V_5–V_6 and, sometimes, V_4.

BIFASCICULAR BLOCK

- Left anterior hemiblock *and* right bundle branch block (see above).

SUPRAVENTRICULAR RHYTHMS

COMMON SUPRAVENTRICULAR RHYTHMS

- Sinus rhythm.
- Atrial extrasystoles.
- Junctional (AV nodal) extrasystoles.
- Atrial tachycardia.
- Atrial flutter.
- Junctional (AV nodal) tachycardia.
- Junctional (AV nodal) escape.
- Atrial fibrillation.

RHYTHM ABNORMALITIES

- Extrasystoles: single early beats suppressing the next sinus beat.
- Escape beats: absence of sinus beat followed by late single beat.
- Tachycardias.
- Bradycardias.

- Ventricular extrasystoles:
  — early QRS complex
  — no P wave
  — QRS complex wide (greater than 120 ms)
  — abnormally shaped QRS complex
  — abnormally shaped T wave
  — next P wave is on time.
- Accelerated idioventricular rhythm.
- Ventricular escape (single beats or complete heart block).
- Ventricular tachycardia:
  — no P waves
  — QRS complex rate greater than 160/min
  — accelerated idioventricular rhythm: as for ventricular tachycardia, but QRS complex rate less than 120/min.
- Ventricular fibrillation:
  — look at the patient, not the ECG.

MYOCARDIAL INFARCTION

SEQUENCE OF ECG CHANGES

1. Normal ECG.
2. Raised ST segments.
3. Appearance of Q waves.
4. Normalization of ST segments.
5. Inversion of T waves.

SITE OF INFARCTION

- Anterior infarction: changes classically in leads V_3–V_4, but often also in leads V_2 and V_5.
- Inferior infarction: changes in leads III and VF.
- Lateral infarction: changes in leads I, VL, V_5–V_6.
- True posterior infarction: dominant R waves in lead V_1.

PULMONARY EMBOLISM

Possible ECG patterns include:

- Normal ECG with sinus tachycardia.
- Peaked P waves.
- Right axis deviation.
- Right bundle branch block.
- Dominant R waves in lead V_1 (i.e. R wave bigger than S wave).
- Inverted T waves in leads V_1–V_3.
- Deep S waves in lead V_6.
- Right axis deviation (S waves in lead I), plus Q waves and inverted T waves in lead III.

HYPERTROPHY OF THE HEART

RIGHT VENTRICULAR HYPERTROPHY

- Right axis deviation.
- Tall R waves in lead V_1.
- T wave inversion in leads V_1–V_2, and sometimes in V_3 and even V_4.
- Deep S waves in lead V_6.
- Sometimes, right bundle branch block.

LEFT VENTRICULAR HYPERTROPHY

- R waves in lead V_5 or V_6 greater than 25 mm.
- R waves in lead V_5 or V_6 plus S waves in lead V_1 or V_2 greater than 35 mm.
- Inverted T waves in leads I, VL, V_5–V_6 and, sometimes, V_4.

LEFT ATRIAL HYPERTROPHY

- Bifid P waves.

RIGHT ATRIAL HYPERTROPHY

- Peaked P waves.

DIFFERENTIAL DIAGNOSIS OF ECG CHANGES

We can rearrange some of these lists to remind you of the possible implications of ECG patterns.

P:QRS APPARENTLY NOT 1:1

If you cannot see one P wave per QRS complex, consider the following:

1. P wave is actually present but not easily visible: look particularly at leads II and V_1.
2. If QRS complexes are irregular, the rhythm is probably atrial fibrillation and what seem to be P waves actually are not.
3. If the QRS complex rate is rapid and there are no P waves, a wide QRS complex indicates ventricular tachycardia and a narrow QRS complex indicates junctional (AV nodal) tachycardia.
4. If the QRS complex rate is slow, it is probably an escape rhythm.

P:QRS MORE THAN 1:1

If you can see more P waves than QRS complexes, consider the following:

1. If the P wave rate is 300/min, the rhythm is atrial flutter.
2. If the P wave rate is 150–200/min and there are two P waves per QRS complex, the rhythm is atrial tachycardia with block.
3. If the P wave rate is normal (i.e. 60–100/min) and there is 2:1 conduction, the rhythm is sinus with second degree block.
4. If the PR interval appears to be different with each beat, complete (third degree) heart block is probably present.

WIDE QRS COMPLEXES (GREATER THAN 120 ms)

Wide QRS complexes are characteristic of:

- Sinus rhythm with bundle branch block.
- Sinus rhythm with the Wolff–Parkinson–White syndrome.
- Ventricular extrasystoles.
- Ventricular tachycardia.
- Complete heart block.

Q WAVES

- Small (septal) Q waves are normal in leads I, VL and V_6.
- Q wave in lead III but not VF is a normal variant.
- Probably indicate infarction if present in more than one lead, longer than 40 ms in duration, and deeper than 2 mm.
- Q waves in lead III but not in VF, plus right axis deviation, may indicate pulmonary embolism.
- Leads showing Q waves indicate site of infarction.

ST SEGMENT DEPRESSION

- Digoxin: ST segment slopes downwards.
- Ischaemia: flat ST segment depression.

T WAVE INVERSION

- Normal in leads III, VR, V_1 and V_2, and in V_3 in black people.
- Ventricular rhythms.
- Bundle branch block.
- Myocardial infarction.
- Right or left ventricular hypertrophy.
- The Wolff–Parkinson–White syndrome.

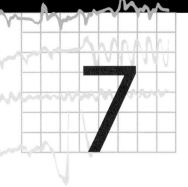

7

Now test yourself

You should now be able to recognize the common ECG patterns, and this final chapter contains ten 12-lead records for you to interpret. But do not forget two important things: first, an ECG comes from an individual patient and must be interpreted with the patient in mind, and second, there is little point in recording and interpreting an ECG unless you are prepared to take some action based on your findings. This is a theme developed in the companion to this book, *150 ECG Problems*. With each of the following ECGs there is a short clinical scenario, and with the interpretation comes a brief suggestion for action.

When reporting an ECG, remember:

- The ECG is easy.
- A report has two parts – a description and an interpretation.
- Look at all the leads, and describe the ECG in the same order every time:
  - rhythm
  - conduction
  - PR interval if sinus rhythm
  - cardiac axis
  - QRS complexes:
    - duration
    - height of R and S waves
    - presence of Q waves
  - ST segments
  - T waves.
- The range of normality, and especially which leads can show an inverted T wave in a normal ECG.

Then, and only then, make a diagnosis.

The ten ECGs here are in no particular sequence, but all have been described earlier in this book. Their descriptions and interpretations are given after the final ECG, commencing on p. 158.

ECG 1

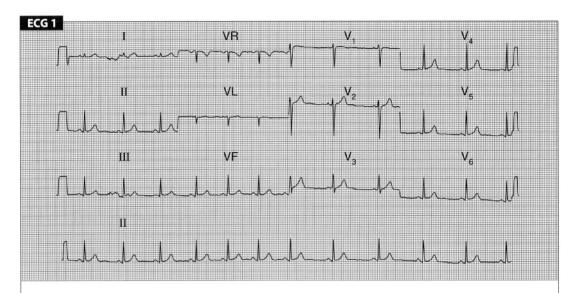

This ECG was recorded from a 20-year-old female medical student who complained of vague chest pain, which she had had intermittently for several months. It was unpredictable, though she thought it might occur at the end of a day when she had been unusually physically active. It lasted for hours at a time. It was not immediately related to activity, nor was it affected by emotional stress, food, or cold weather. It was relieved by paracetamol. On examination there were no abnormalities.

ECG 2

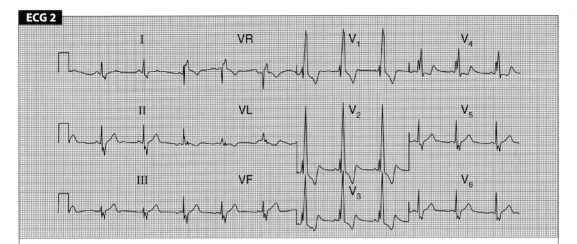

This ECG was recorded from an 18-year-old student nurse who had been found to have a heart murmur at a routine medical examination. She thought that it had also been heard during school medical examinations, but no action had been taken. She had no symptoms. On examination her heart was regular, there was no clinical evidence of cardiac enlargement, and there was a moderately loud ejection systolic murmur at the left sternal edge. This murmur became louder on inspiration. The pulmonary second sound was widely split, with no variation on respiration.

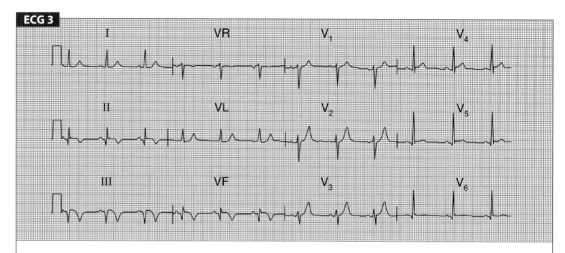

ECG 3

A 60-year-old man was sent to hospital by his GP because he had had severe central chest pain 48 h earlier. The pain had lasted about 3 h. Previously he had been well, and by the time he was seen he was pain-free and there were no abnormalities on examination.

ECG 4

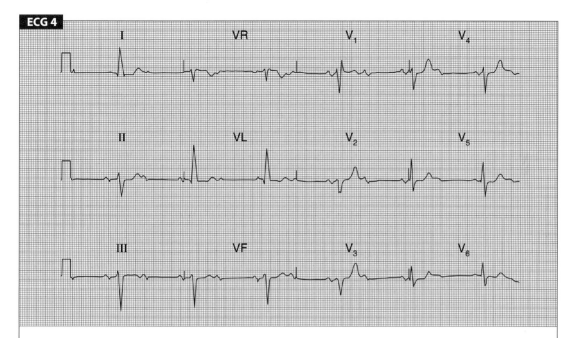

An 80-year-old woman complained of attacks of dizziness for the past year. These were infrequent but could come on at any time, without obvious precipitating events, and they could occur whether she was standing or lying down. She had never had any chest pain, and apart from these attacks she was very well and fully active. Physical examination revealed a regular heart with a rate of about 40/min, but no other abnormalities.

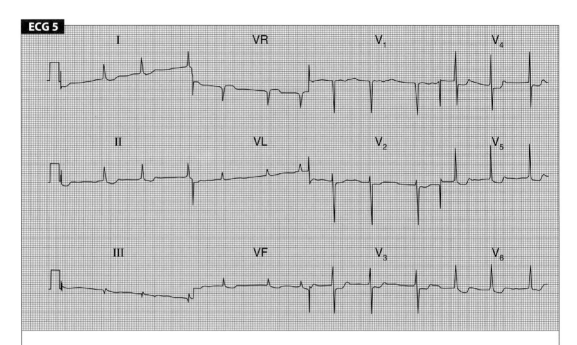

ECG 5

This is an ECG from a 70-year-old woman whose main complaint was lethargy. For the past year she had been breathless and had had some ankle swelling, and she had been taking tablets for this. She felt sick and had lost a little weight. Physical examination revealed an irregular pulse and signs of mild heart failure.

ECG 6

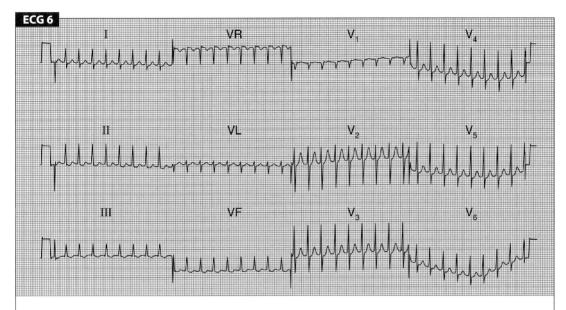

A 25-year-old man presented to the A & E department complaining of severe palpitations for 2 h. He had had occasional such attacks since he was a teenager, but no ECG had been recorded. A typical attack would begin suddenly and stop suddenly after a variable period. During the attack he would often feel breathless and a little dizzy. On examination he looked well, and apart from a heart rate of 170/min and a blood pressure of 90/70 there were no abnormalities.

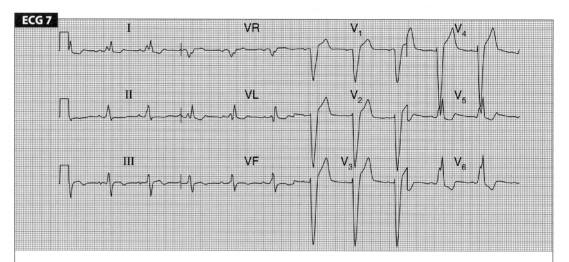

ECG 7

This ECG was recorded from a 60-year-old orthopaedic surgeon who said that whenever he climbed a certain hill on his golf course, he had a sensation of pressure across the front of his chest, and he felt dizzy. This had happened for about 6 months, and he had never had any problems at any other time. On examination his heart was regular, his blood pressure was 110/90, and there was a systolic murmur which could be heard all over the front of the chest but which was loudest at the upper right sternal edge. It radiated into the neck.

ECG 8

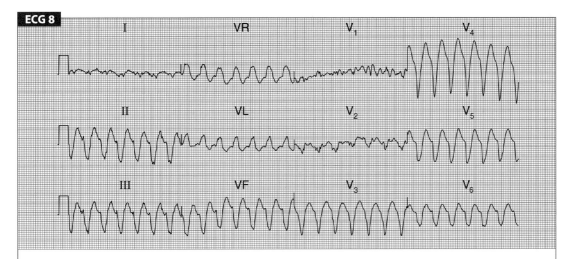

A 50-year-old man who was in a coronary care unit recovering from an acute myocardial infarction suddenly complained of palpitations, breathlessness and chest pain. His heart rate was 160/min, his blood pressure was 90/60 and he had signs of pulmonary oedema.

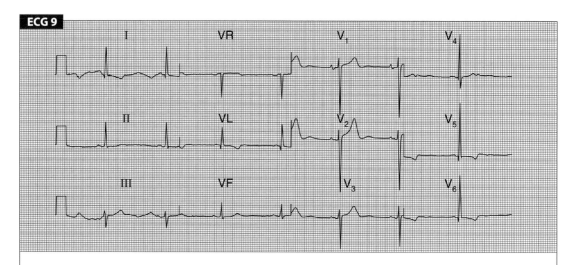

ECG 9

A 30-year-old man was found at a routine examination to have a blood pressure of 220/120. He had no symptoms. He had not been examined for many years, and it was not clear how long his blood pressure had been so high. On examination his cardiac apex beat was displaced to the anterior axillary line in the sixth rib interspace. The pulses in his legs were difficult to feel.

ECG 10

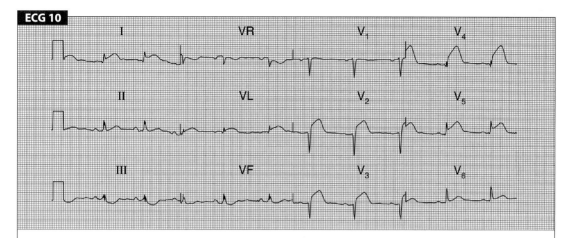

This ECG was recorded from a 50-year-old man who was admitted to hospital with severe central chest pain which he had had for 1 h. He had been a heavy smoker for many years. He described the pain as heavy, and continuous; it was central and radiated through to the back. It was not affected by respiration or position. On examination his skin felt cold and sweaty, but his blood pressure was normal and all his peripheral pulses were palpable. There were no cardiac murmurs.

ECG DESCRIPTIONS AND INTERPRETATIONS

ECG 1

This ECG shows:

- Sinus rhythm; rhythm strip (lead II) shows sinus arrhythmia
- Normal PR interval, 120 ms
- Normal axis
- QRS complex duration 80 ms, normal height
- ST segment isoelectric in all leads
- T wave inversion in lead VR, but no other lead

Interpretation of the ECG

This is a perfectly normal record in all respects. The sinus arrhythmia is clearly shown in the section of the rhythm strip shown below: the change in R–R interval is progressive from beat to beat, and the configuration of the P wave does not change, so there is sinus rhythm throughout.

If you did not get this right, look again at pp. 65–66.

Rhythm strip

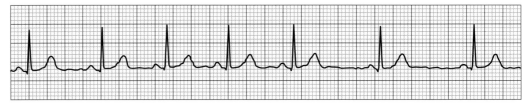

Clinical management

The description of the pain does not sound in the least cardiac, and a young woman is very unlikely to have coronary disease anyway. If you find yourself making a diagnosis on the basis of the ECG that seems clinically unlikely, think about the ECG a little further. This pain sounds muscular, and she only needs reassurance.

ECG
IP

For more information on normal variants of the ECG, see p. 49

ECG 2

This ECG shows:

- Sinus rhythm
- Normal PR interval
- Normal axis
- Wide QRS complex duration, at 160 ms
- RSR[1] pattern in lead V_1
- Wide and notched S wave in lead V_6
- ST segment isoelectric
- T wave inversion in lead VR (normal), and in leads V_1–V_3

Interpretation of the ECG

There is no problem with conduction between the atria and the ventricles because the PR interval is normal and constant. The prolonged QRS complex duration shows that there is conduction delay within the ventricles. The RSR[1] pattern in lead V_1 and the deep and wide S wave in lead V_6 (see extracts from traces, below) are characteristic of right bundle branch block (RBBB).

Any problems? If so, look at pp. 49–51.

V_1

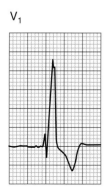

V_6

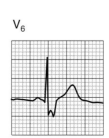

Clinical management

The story raises the possibility that this young woman has a congenital heart problem. An ejection systolic murmur at the left sternal edge, which becomes louder on inspiration, suggests a pulmonary murmur. Fixed wide splitting of the second heart sound is the clinical manifestation of RBBB, with which pulmonary valve closure is delayed. RBBB is characteristic of an atrial septal defect, and an echocardiogram is essential to confirm the diagnosis and help decide if, how, and when it should be closed.

For more information on congenital heart disease, see p. 257

ECG 3

This ECG shows:

- Sinus rhythm
- Normal PR interval
- Normal axis
- QRS complex has Q waves in leads II, III, VF
- ST segment isoelectric
- T waves inverted in leads II, III, VF

Interpretation of the ECG

The Q waves in leads III and VF, together with the inverted T waves in those leads (see extract from trace, below), indicate an inferior myocardial infarction. Since the ST segment is virtually isoelectric (i.e.

III

VF

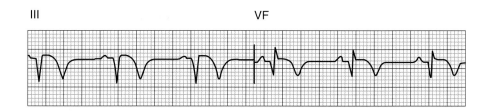

at baseline, and not elevated) the infarction is 'old'. The ECG can show this pattern at any time after the 24 h following the infarction, so timing the event is not possible from the ECG.

Get this one wrong? Read pp. 111–113.

Clinical management

The clinical story suggests that the infarction occurred 48 h previously. This patient has presented too late for immediate treatment of the infarction by thrombolysis or urgent angioplasty, and he does not need pain relief or any treatment for complications. The aim of management is therefore to prevent a further infarction and he will need long-term aspirin, a beta-blocker, an ACE inhibitor and a statin. He will also need an exercise test and a decision will need to be made about the need for coronary angiography.

For more information on myocardial infarction, see p. 165

ECG 4

This ECG shows:

- Sinus rhythm
- Alternate conducted and non-conducted beats
- Normal PR interval in the conducted beats
- Left axis deviation (deep S waves in leads II and III)
- Wide QRS complex (duration 160 ms)
- RSR^1 pattern in lead V_1

Interpretation of the ECG

The alternating conducted and non-conducted P waves indicate second degree heart block, and this explains the slow heart rate. The left axis deviation shows that conduction down the anterior fascicle of the left bundle branch is blocked, and the RSR^1 pattern in lead V_1 indicates right bundle branch block (see extracts from traces, overleaf).

This was explained on p. 48.

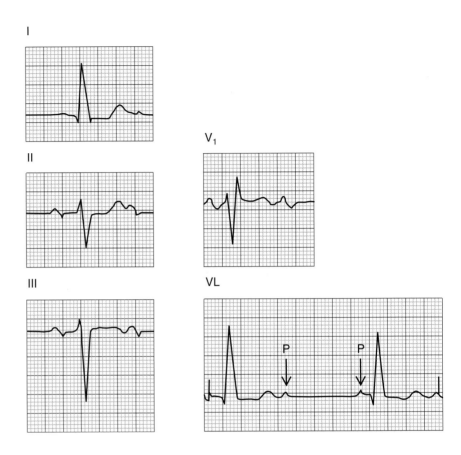

I

II

V₁

III

VL

P ↓   P ↓

Clinical management

This patient clearly has severe disease of her conduction system. Both bundle branches are affected, and the second degree block probably results from disease in the His bundle. The attacks of dizziness may be due to further slowing of the heart rate with the same rhythm, or may be due to intermittent complete heart block (Stokes–Adams attacks). This could be investigated with a 24-h ambulatory ECG recording, but this is not really necessary as she needs an immediate permanent pacemaker.

ECG
IP

For more information on pacemakers, see

p. 283

ECG 5

The ECG shows:

- Atrial fibrillation
- Normal axis
- Normal QRS complexes
- Downward-sloping ST segments, best seen in leads V_4–V_6
- U waves, best seen in lead V_2

Interpretation of the ECG

The completely irregular rhythm with narrow QRS complexes must be due to atrial fibrillation, even though the usual baseline irregularity is not very obvious. The downward-sloping ST segments indicate that she is taking digoxin, which explains the good control of the ventricular rate (with untreated atrial fibrillation the ventricular rate would usually be rapid), and the U waves suggest hypokalaemia (see extracts from traces, below: in lead V_5, the downward-sloping ST segment is arrowed).

If you made a mistake with this one, read p. 114.

V_2

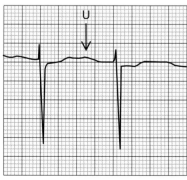

V_5

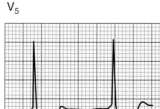

Clinical management

If this patient who is taking digoxin feels sick, she is probably suffering from digoxin toxicity, and hypokalaemia may be the main cause of this. Hypokalaemia is likely to occur if a patient with heart failure is given a loop diuretic without either a potassium-retaining diuretic or potassium supplements. The serum potassium must be checked urgently, and appropriate action taken.

Remember that we have still not made a full diagnosis: what is the cause of the atrial fibrillation? Most cardiac conditions can be associated with atrial fibrillation, but in elderly patients the important disease to remember is thyrotoxicosis, because atrial fibrillation may be the only manifestation of this in the elderly.

For more information on electrolyte abnormalities, see p. 267

ECG 6

This ECG shows:

- Narrow QRS complexes (duration less than 120 ms)
- Tachycardia at 200/min
- No visible P waves
- QRS complexes normal
- ST segments show a little depression in leads II, III, VF
- T waves normal except in lead III

Interpretation of the ECG

The QRS complexes are narrow, so this is a supraventricular tachycardia. It is regular, so it is not atrial fibrillation. No P waves are visible, so it is not sinus rhythm, atrial tachycardia or atrial flutter (see extract from trace, opposite). This has to be an AV nodal re-entry, or junctional, rhythm (sometimes, but not logically, referred to as 'supraventricular tachycardia'). The clinical story would be entirely consistent with episodes of this arrhythmia.

In case of difficulty, look at pp. 81–82.

V_3

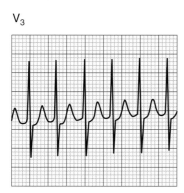

Clinical management

This rhythm can often be terminated by carotid sinus pressure, or by the Valsalva manoeuvre. Failing that, it will usually respond to intravenous adenosine. DC cardioversion should be considered for any patient with a tachycardia that is compromising the circulation. The best way of preventing the attacks depends on their frequency and severity. An electrophysiological study, with a view to possible ablation of an abnormal conducting pathway, should be considered.

For more information on electrophysiology and ablation, see p. 314

ECG 7

This ECG shows:

- Sinus rhythm
- Normal PR interval
- Normal axis
- Wide QRS complexes, duration 200 ms
- 'M' pattern in leads I, VL, V_5–V_6
- Deep S waves in leads V_2–V_4
- Biphasic or inverted T waves in leads I, VL V_5–V_6

Interpretation of the ECG

The rhythm and PR interval are normal but the wide QRS complexes show that there is a conduction delay within the ventricles. The 'M' pattern, best seen in the lateral leads (see extract from lead V$_6$, below) shows that this is left bundle branch block (LBBB). In LBBB the T waves are usually inverted in the lateral leads, and have no further significance. In the presence of LBBB the ECG cannot be interpreted any further, so it is not possible to comment on the presence or absence of ischaemia.

If you need to check, look at pp. 51–53 and 55.

V$_6$

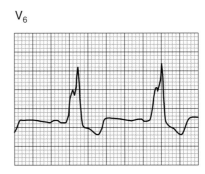

Clinical management

The story sounds like angina, but when angina is combined with dizziness always think of aortic stenosis, which can also cause angina even with normal coronary arteries. This is what the physical signs suggest. LBBB is common in aortic stenosis. A patient with aortic stenosis who is dizzy on exertion has a high risk of sudden death, and this patient needs urgent investigation with a view to early aortic valve replacement.

ECG
IP

For more information on the ECG in patients with dizziness, see p. 61

ECG 8

This ECG shows:

- Broad complex tachycardia at 160/min
- No P waves visible
- Left axis deviation
- QRS complex duration 200 ms
- QRS complexes all point downwards in the chest leads
- Artefacts in leads I, V_1–V_2

Interpretation of the ECG

The QRS complexes are broad, so this is either a ventricular tachycardia or a supraventricular tachycardia with bundle branch block. There are no P waves, so it is not sinus rhythm or an atrial rhythm. The QRS complexes are regular, so it is not atrial fibrillation, but an AV nodal rhythm with bundle branch block has to be a possibility. However, the left axis deviation, and the 'concordance' of the QRS complexes (all pointing downwards), makes this ventricular tachycardia (see extracts from traces, below).

The diagnosis of tachycardias is covered on p. 77.

II

III

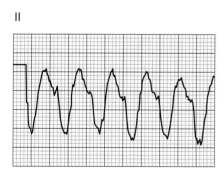
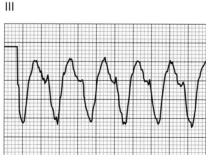

For more information on the differentiation of broad complex tachycardias, see p. 111

Clinical management

In the context of a myocardial infarction, a broad complex tachycardia is almost always ventricular in origin and there is no need to get too puzzled by the ECG. This patient has developed pulmonary oedema, so needs urgent treatment. While preparations are made for DC cardioversion he could be given intravenous lignocaine and furosemide, but you should not rely on a satisfactory response to drug therapy.

ECG 9

This ECG shows:

- Sinus rhythm
- Bifid P waves
- Normal conducting intervals
- Normal axis
- Tall R wave in lead V_5 and deep S wave in lead V_2
- Small (septal) Q wave in leads I, VL, V_5–V_6
- Inverted T waves in leads I, VL, V_5–V_6
- U waves in leads V_2–V_4 (normal)

Interpretation of the ECG

The bifid P waves, best seen in lead V_3, indicate left atrial hypertrophy (see extracts from trace, opposite). The combined height of the R wave in lead V_5 plus the depth of the S wave in lead V_2 is 58 mm, so there are 'voltage criteria' for left ventricular hypertrophy. The inverted T waves in the lateral leads confirm severe left ventricular hypertrophy. The Q waves are small and narrow, and are therefore septal in origin and do not indicate an old infarction.

If you needed help with this one, re-read pp. 102 and 103.

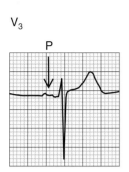

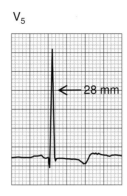

Clinical management

This patient has clinical and ECG evidence of left ventricular hypertrophy, but this is not a full diagnosis – what might be the cause of the hypertension? A young man with hypertension who has abnormal pulses in the legs almost certainly has a coarctation of the aorta, which needs investigation and correction.

For more information on the diagnosis of left ventricular hypertrophy, see p. 235

ECG 10

This ECG shows:

- Sinus rhythm
- Normal conducting intervals
- Normal axis
- Small R waves in leads V_1–V_2
- Very small R wave in lead V_3
- Small Q wave and very small R wave in lead V_4
- Raised ST segments in leads I, VL, V_2–V_5

Interpretation of the ECG

The small R waves in leads V_1–V_2 could be normal, but leads V_3–V_4 should show larger R waves. The raised ST segments indicate an ST segment elevation myocardial infarction (see extracts from traces, below). The small Q wave in lead V_4 suggests that a fairly short time has elapsed since the onset of the infarction, and this Q wave will probably become larger over the next few hours. Since the changes are limited to leads I, VL and V_2–V_5, this is an acute anterolateral myocardial infarction.

You must have got this one right – the ECG is easy!

V_3 V_4

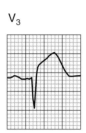
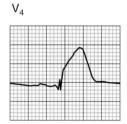

For more information on myocardial infarction, see p. 165

If you find testing yourself helpful, try *150 ECG Problems*.

Clinical management

This man needs urgent pain relief. Pain radiating to the back always raises the possibility of an aortic dissection, but it is quite common in acute infarction and there are no physical signs – loss of pulses, asymmetric blood pressure in the arms, a murmur of aortic regurgitation or pericarditis – to support a diagnosis of aortic dissection. If in doubt an urgent echocardiogram may help, but essentially this patient needs either immediate thrombolysis or angioplasty.

The moral of this story – and of all the others – is that an ECG is an aid to diagnosis, not a substitute for further thought.

Index

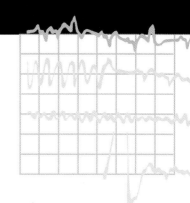

Note: Page numbers in **bold** refer to figures and tables.
Abbreviations used in subentries: LBBB, left bundle branch block; RBBB, right bundle branch block.